Par

Healthy
Neurodevelopment

Stewarding Your Child's Brain
From Conception to Graduation

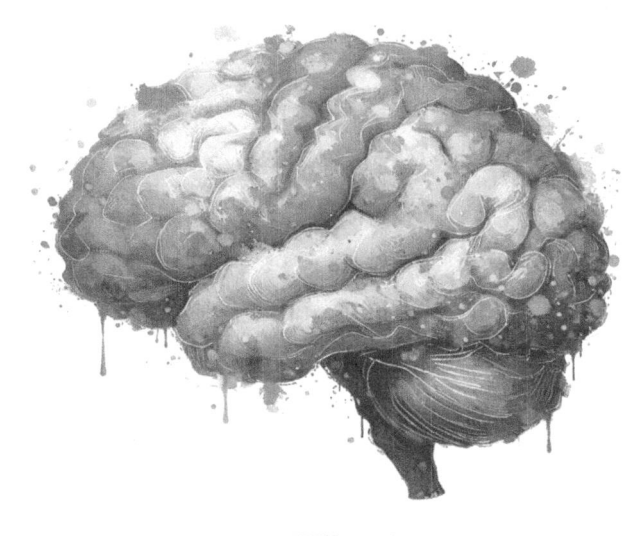

DR. CHRIS SLININGER, DC, DCCJP
DR. ETHAN SURPRENANT, DC

Parent's Guide to Healthy Neurodevelopment

Published by the Authors
https://DrChrisSlininger.com

ISBN
Paperback: 979-8-9933154-0-9

First Edition, 2025

Medical Disclaimer
The information in this book is provided for educational purposes only and is not medical advice. It is not intended to diagnose, treat, cure, or prevent any disease, and it does not create a doctor–patient relationship. Always seek the advice of your physician, pediatrician, or other qualified health provider with any questions you may have regarding a medical condition. Never disregard professional medical advice or delay seeking it because of something you have read in this book. If you believe your child may be experiencing a medical emergency, call your local emergency number immediately.

Cover design, interior design, and illustrations by Dr. Chris Slininger
Photo credits: Dr. Chris Slininger

Printed in the United States of America by Amazon KDP

Table of Contents

Introduction

A Message from Dr. Chris Slininger

I've always dreamed of helping the everyday family have a better understanding of what causes the body to be healthy. I grew up in a house where we did our best, but the truth is we just didn't have a lot of knowledge about what made the body truly well. I don't think it was anyone's fault—it's simply all we knew, and we did the best we could with what we had.

But over time, after going to doctor after doctor and asking question after question about what was causing illnesses and issues, the answers my family received were so poor and unsatisfying that something was planted deep inside me. It created a burning desire to find out for myself: not just what caused sickness, but what made the body well at its very core.

As a teenager, I started chasing those answers. Much of it was experimentation—putting my own body to the test just to see what would happen. When I got to undergrad, I majored in athletic training. I learned a lot about physical fitness, injury prevention, and rehabilitation, but the bigger questions were still there. Why was the body breaking down in the first place? What made it tick at its deepest level? What really allowed it to thrive?

It wasn't until I met a chiropractor who explained the founding principles of the profession that something clicked. I began to understand that the brain is at the center of it all—that it coordinates every single function of the body through the nervous system, and that any interference in that communication will disrupt health. For the first time, I felt like I'd found an answer that made sense.

So I entered chiropractic school still carrying that seed, determined to get to the bottom of what makes the body well. And as I studied, the veil began to lift. I started to grasp the principles of what allows the brain and body to function at their absolute best. But even then, I didn't stop—I pushed further into postgraduate work because I wanted more than just a partial answer. I wanted it to make sense, and I wanted to be able to explain it in a way that others could truly grasp.

And that's where this book comes in. One of my deepest passions has always been to take complicated science and make it simple. If it can't be explained plainly—through stories, analogies, and everyday language—then it's not very useful for the people who need it most: families. Even doctors learn best through stories and simple principles, so how much more do parents deserve to have these truths made accessible?

This book is the culmination of what Dr. Ethan Surprenant and I have been able to learn, live, and now share in a way that makes sense for everyday families. Together, we want to give you a 10,000-foot view of neurodevelopment—an overview of the anatomy, physiology, and developmental concepts that govern how a child's brain grows and matures into adulthood. This isn't a scientific textbook and it's not meant to drown you in research citations. It's meant to give you clarity about the big picture: what makes the brain develop right, what can go wrong, and how you as a parent can steward your child's development in a healthier direction.

I'm honored to write this with Dr. Surprenant. I've seen his heart for families firsthand—especially for parents who feel like they've run into brick walls trying to make sense of their children's struggles. We both share the same passion: bringing health education back into the home. Mothers, fathers, grandparents, and even young couples who haven't yet had children deserve to know these principles.

We live in a culture where medications are often the first resort, but while they may mask symptoms, they rarely get to the root. Parents deserve better answers, and kids deserve healthier futures. This book is meant to be a starting point for families who want to go deeper, who want to understand the "why" behind their child's development.

We want your family to be healthier than the last generation, and for your children to grow up with access to knowledge that many of us never had. Our hope is that these principles will not only guide your family now, but will ripple into your children's children as they carry these truths forward.

May this book be a blessing to your family, to your children, and to generations yet to come.

Chapter 1

The Role and Function of the Brain

Dr. Chris

The Florida sunlight poured through the windows of our small bungalow in St. Petersburg, casting a warm glow across the living room. My wife, Mary, and I had just moved across the country from California, settling into a new life after I started working at a clinic nearby. We were still filling our house with furniture and decorations. Our firstborn, Ethan, was playing on one of the first pieces of furniture we'd picked up for the space.

Ethan, our son, was always full of energy—a whirlwind of motion and curiosity. He had this way of attacking the world head-on, always testing limits, always pushing boundaries. That day, he was bouncing on the wide cushions of the sofa. Mary and I kept a watchful eye on him as he leapt from one side to the other, but you could never really contain Ethan. He had a spark in his eyes that seemed too big for his small body, as if his adventurous spirit was constantly at odds with the physical limits of childhood.

Then it happened. We looked away—just for a moment—and when we glanced back, Ethan was mid-lunge, launching himself off the sofa. Except this time, instead of landing on the cushions, he went headfirst toward the floor. His neck bent sharply on impact, and his body crumpled in a way that made me freeze.

The thud was loud, sickening even. He started crying immediately, and Mary rushed to scoop him up, holding him close, trying to comfort him. At first, it seemed like a typical fall—one of those bumps that might scare a child more than hurt them. But this time, something was different.

I leaned in to check on him, my mind racing. Ethan was crying, but as I looked closer, I realized it wasn't the same. His spark was gone.

Even as tears streamed down his face, there was a strange emptiness in his expression. It wasn't the raw emotion of a child who'd been startled or hurt. It felt... detached. He cried, but without the urgency or life I'd come to expect from him. I couldn't shake the feeling that this was no ordinary fall.

Thankfully, I had seen this before—sometimes in kids, often in adults. I knew immediately there was something wrong with the way Ethan's brain was communicating with the rest of his body. And I knew it had to do with his neck.

"Mary, we need to go," I said, gently but firmly. "Load him into the car."

She looked at me, clearly upset, but she trusted me. We couldn't just hold him and hope for the best. He needed help—and it wasn't going to be found at the hospital. Instead, we drove straight to my clinic.

When we arrived, I carried him inside and laid him carefully on the treatment table. His crying had softened to a whimper by then, but the vacant look in his eyes lingered, and it tore at me. I started a series of gentle neurological tests, and what I found confirmed my suspicion: the impact had misaligned his upper neck. That misalignment was creating a big disconnect between his brain and its ability to communicate with the rest of his body. It was also affecting several cranial nerves, which I could see in his dilated pupils. His nervous system wasn't working the way it should.

I moved quickly but deliberately. I laid him down on a specialized adjustment table designed just for kids, then grabbed a percussive sound wave adjusting instrument. Carefully, I positioned it, aimed, and with a precise click, made the adjustment.

Then I squatted down so I was eye level with Ethan, watching and waiting. Five seconds passed. Then ten. It felt like minutes, though I know it wasn't.

And then, suddenly, Ethan took the deepest breath I've ever seen. It was as if he were sucking life back into his body—a gasp so profound it made me hold my own breath. Within moments, his little body relaxed. His pupils began to normalize, his face softened, and he looked... alive again.

I ran another series of tests. Everything came back clear. The connection had been restored. But what mattered most wasn't the data on the tests—it was the spark in Ethan's eyes. He was back. His life, his energy, his Ethan-ness had returned, and as parents, Mary and I both felt an overwhelming sense of relief and gratitude.

We sat there with him for a few minutes, holding him close. Then we loaded him into the car for the short drive home. He fell asleep almost instantly—peaceful, calm, and restored.

That day left a mark on me. It was the first time one of my own children had experienced nerve interference. And while Ethan had only suffered for a few minutes, it struck me how many kids live with this kind of issue for years. As both a parent and a doctor, it made me realize that every parent needs to know what I knew that day—how to restore their child's Neurological Clarity so they can experience the full health and well-being they are designed for...both in their bodies and their brains.

What Does the Brain Do?

What I saw on my son's face that day was more than just a look. As a parent, I felt the gut-wrenching fear of something being wrong. But as a doctor, I immediately recognized the deeper issue: the sudden disconnect between Ethan's brain and his body.

The signs were clear to me. His cranial nerves—the ones that come directly from the brainstem—weren't functioning properly. His cognitive processes were disrupted, and his limbic system, the emotional center of his brain, was compromised. All of this had happened simultaneously in a matter of seconds.

The brain is more than just another organ—it's the body's command center. Every action, every emotion, every movement your child makes starts in the brain. Waking or sleeping, the brain is working nonstop to make your body function.

Different parts of the brain are responsible for specific functions. One area controls movement, while another handles sensation. Some regions interpret what you see, hear, and taste, while others govern speech or regulate emotions. Together, these sections form a living, breathing supercomputer, capable of processing enormous amounts of information from the body and commanding millions of tiny actions at once—all without you ever thinking about it.

But the brain doesn't work alone. It's part of a larger system: the nervous system, which includes the brain, brainstem, spinal cord, and all the nerves that run through the body. This system is the network that links every part of your child's body back to their brain, ensuring constant communication and coordination.

What's fascinating is how interconnected the brain and body are. The body expresses outwardly what the brain decides internally. If the brain is sending the wrong messages—or no messages at all—you'll see the effects almost immediately in how the body responds. In Ethan's case, his fall caused a misalignment in his neck, disrupting communication between his brain and his body. That miscommunication was visible in everything from his pupils to his posture.

Despite its critical role, the nervous system is often overlooked. Think about this: when you take your child to the pediatrician for a checkup, they'll evaluate many of the body's systems. The doctor will listen to the heart, check the lungs, and even review the digestive and endocrine systems. But what about the central nervous system—the system responsible for coordinating all of the others?

At most, the doctor might test a knee reflex or a few cranial nerve tests, but there's rarely a thorough evaluation of how well the nervous system is carrying out its role. Things like balance, coordination, and limbic system function are usually overlooked. This has always struck me as odd. If the brain controls all of the body's other systems, wouldn't it make sense to check its function first?

The truth is, problems in the nervous system often go unnoticed for years. Children can adapt to miscommunications within the brain-body connection, making it harder to spot subtle issues. But those problems don't go away. They grow, affecting everything from physical health to emotional resilience and even cognitive development. That's why understanding what the brain does—and how to ensure it's working properly—is the cornerstone of ensuring healthy neurodevelopment.

The Purpose of This Guide

The reason Dr. Ethan and I created this guide is simple: we want to give every parent the tools they need to build strong foundations for their kids, no matter their stage of development. Throughout the book, Dr. Ethan and I will take turns sharing.

When my son was injured that day, I had the privilege of knowing exactly what to do. I had to, as I like to put it, "turn his power back on." But here's the truth—without my training, I likely would have taken him to the hospital or our pediatrician. While those seem to be reasonable steps most people, they wouldn't have addressed the root issue because the signs and symptoms of nervous system dysfunction are often subtle or misunderstood. My background gave me the ability to spot the problem and fix it, and it's that knowledge we want to share with you in this guide.

This book is meant to be a tool—a practical, straightforward reference for parents. We understand you don't have much time. You don't need an entire novel about parenting. What you do need is a clear, easy-to-follow resource, with relatable stories, that highlight the most important principles of healthy neurodevelopment.

Why principles? Because principles outlast trends and techniques. I think Ralph Waldo Emerson said it best:

> *"As to the methods, there may be a million and then some, but principles are few. The man who grasps principles can successfully select his own methods. The man who tries methods, ignoring principles, is sure to have trouble."*

Much of today's parenting advice is built around methods—tips, systems, and quick fixes that flood social media and parenting articles. You can scroll endlessly and find a strategy for almost any situation, but the sheer volume is often more confusing than helpful. Without a clear sense of the principles beneath it all—what children truly need and how their bodies are designed to function—it's easy to feel overwhelmed and end up choosing solutions that only cover surface problems.

This guide is built on key principles that we call the Six Pillars of Health. These foundational ideas will give you an understanding of how your child's body —and your own—functions. By mastering these principles, you'll gain the clarity and confidence to make thoughtful decisions, even when unexpected challenges arise. It allows you to get below the surface and become an excellent steward of your child's neurodevelopment.

It's the same clarity that allowed me to act decisively for my son that day—to restore the spark of life to his body. That's what I want for every child: to have and keep that spark and to grow up with a strong foundation for health and well-being.

Let's dive into the Six Pillars of Health.

Chapter 2

The Six Pillars of Health

Building Firm Foundations

Dr. Chris

For the past 16 years, I have had the privilege of teaching courses on anatomy, physiology, neurology, and a variety of other health topics ranging from nutrition and exercise to health-specific webinars. Teaching has always been a passion of mine, but for years, I felt like something was missing.

The courses I taught were often fragmented. Each one focused on a specific area, and while the information was valuable, the big picture was missing. People were walking away with pieces of the puzzle but without a way to put them together. That really concerned me. They needed to see the whole puzzle put together.

The turning point came after a conversation with my wife, Mary. She'd seen me teach class after class for different audiences, and one day, she pointed out something that stuck with me: "People need categories to put the information in. Without that, it's just scattered bits of knowledge."

At first, I resisted the idea. As someone who studies the human body, I know it's far too dynamic and interconnected to be limited to a few categories. But Mary was right—without a framework to organize the information, it's hard for anyone to understand how it all fits together.

That realization started me on a journey. I began praying for guidance, asking God to show me how to make this information not only more cohesive, but also more practical for people to use in their everyday lives. I wanted a framework that would help people not just understand their health, but apply that understanding to themselves and their families.

Through a mix of counsel, inspiration, and what I believe was God's guidance, I landed on this framework—the Six Pillars of Health. The Six Pillars of Health include Mental Acuity, Emotional Fortitude, Chemical Purity, Nutritional Saturation, Structural Stability, and Neurological Clarity. This structure provides a clear, straightforward way to understand the key principles that underlie health and neurodevelopment. It's simple enough to be accessible, yet deep enough to cover the most important aspects of the human body and mind.

The reason why these categories are so important is not only because they are independently essential for the health of the human body, but also because they are interconnected with each of the other pillars. For example, we start with Mental Acuity because it is so important to have the right perspective about your health in order to make sound-minded decisions. If you are really sick but believe you are healthy, then your starting point is already wrong, and that misunderstanding will influence every choice you make.

But if you can clearly understand how the body is designed to function and where you actually are along the spectrum of health, that accurate perspective gives you the ability to make wise decisions that bring your behaviors and health into good order. Mental Acuity is also the ability to think sharply and intelligently. The clearer we can think, the better decisions we can make—decisions that shape the course of our lives from childhood through old age.

Emotional Fortitude is just as vital. It is very difficult to stay strong and stable if you are easily derailed by outside influences or challenging situations. Emotional Fortitude is about resilience—the ability to make a decision and be tough enough to carry it out, even when life gets hard. I have known many people with incredible intelligence and capacity who still fell short of their goals, not because they lacked ability, but because they lacked discipline or were easily thrown off course by the pressures of life. Emotional Fortitude is not only about inner strength, but also about cultivating peace. When we are steady on the inside, even when circumstances are difficult on the outside, our bodies are able to thrive.

But even if we have the right mindset and the resilience to set goals and pursue them, the body still has essential physical needs. Another essential pillar is Chemical Purity. It is impossible for the body to be toxic and healthy at the same time. Any buildup of toxins—whether from food, environment, or medications—interferes with how the body works and robs it of vitality. This is true for both children and adults, and protecting Chemical Purity is one of the most basic requirements for the body to function as it was designed.

In addition, we need Nutritional Saturation. This is more than just eating a "healthy diet." It's about maximizing the nutrients our bodies take in, because nutrients are the building blocks of life itself. Nutritional Saturation ensures the body has the raw materials it needs to grow, repair, and function properly. This is especially true for children, whose rapidly developing bodies require an abundance of building blocks to construct strong, healthy systems. Without Nutritional Saturation, the body simply cannot perform at its best.

We must also consider Structural Stability. For anything in the body to work well, it must be structurally sound. The bones, joints, and connective tissues have to be strong, well-built, and properly aligned. A weak structure, or one that is misaligned or unstable, will inevitably compromise health and function. Structural Stability is the foundation that allows all other systems to work properly, because without it, the body's design is compromised.

And finally, tying everything together is Neurological Clarity. The nervous system is the master control system of the body, and nothing in the body works without a nerve signal directing it. Neurological Clarity ensures that the communication between brain and body remains free from interference, so that every organ, system, and cell knows exactly what to do and how to do it. When the nervous system is clear, the body can function as it was designed, allowing all the other pillars to operate in harmony.

When we take these Six Pillars—Mental Acuity, Emotional Fortitude, Chemical Purity, Nutritional Saturation, Structural Stability, and Neurological Clarity—and put them together, they become the solid foundation of health. When all six are understood, strengthened, and well-stewarded, the body thrives. If you are a good steward of your health and manage each of these pillars well, your body—or your child's body—becomes far more resilient. It is difficult for the brain to malfunction, for chronic sickness to take hold, or for neurodevelopment to go off track. But if any of these pillars are compromised or neglected, the effects ripple outward, influencing both brain and body in profound ways.

Think of the Six Pillars like the legs of a sturdy table. A table with all six legs firmly in place is stable, durable, and ready to bear weight. But if one leg is wobbly—or worse, missing—the whole table is compromised. In the same way, when any one of these pillars is neglected, the foundation of health begins to erode. The more severe the neglect, the more significant the problem becomes.

In the chapters ahead, we'll begin to unpack each of these Six Pillars—not in exhaustive detail, but enough to help you understand how they support healthy neurodevelopment. As you see the principles behind them more clearly, we'll also weave them into the stages of a child's growth, showing how they remain critical from conception to graduation. The goal is to give you a practical understanding of what's happening at each stage and how you can be a wise steward of these pillars, so that your child's brain and body are equipped to thrive through every stage of development.

Chapter 3

Mental Acuity

A Right Perspective of Your Child's Body

Dr. Chris

As a parent, it's your job to piece together what's happening in your child's body and make decisions that support their long-term well-being. But to do that, you need the right perspective—a clear understanding of how the body works and what it means to be truly healthy.

This is a conversation I have with adults all the time.

They'll come into my office and say, "I'm doing really well. My health is good. My doctor has me on this new medication, and I'm feeling better now."

I'll look at them and gently reply, "You're not well."

They're often surprised, sometimes defensive. "What do you mean? I feel fine!"

That's when I remind them: health is not based on how you feel; it's based on how you function. This common mindset that I frequently encounter is deeply flawed, and it becomes even more dangerous when we apply it to our children.

In the United States, we've been conditioned to believe that the highest form of health is simply the absence of discomfort. If we can suppress a symptom, we think we're healthy. We are bombarded with medications and misinformed about how the body works keeping our society largely ignorant of the foundational principles that make us well.

As parents, it's easy to get overwhelmed when you see your child with fevers, sniffles, stress responses, lack of focus, or low energy. Naturally, parents want their child to feel better, but suppressing symptoms doesn't address the underlying issue. The symptoms are just indicators—like a blinking check engine light on your car.

When the check engine light comes on, you don't cover it with tape and hope for the best. You pop the hood and figure out what's going on underneath. The same principle applies to your child's health. Symptoms are messages from the body, signaling that something needs attention. The goal is to understand the root cause, not just silence the signal.

Unfortunately, many parents equate symptom suppression with health. A child may be on three different medications to manage anxiety, allergies, or other chronic symptoms. Parents can convince themselves that this means their children are fine. But this is actually what I would call delusion. The moment those children stop taking those medication's, the condition is still there waiting for them. This means that the conditions that they are experiencing our active whether or not a child is on a medication.

I know calling this way of thinking delusional is a strong way to put it, but the consequences to our children are so significant if we do not get our mindset right. It is critical that we take the time to understand the underlying issue and the reason why they have the condition in the first place.

Children rely on us to guide their health. They don't yet have a full grasp of how their bodies work or the wisdom to make sound decisions that lead to better outcomes. On top of that, every medical intervention requires a parent's approval. If we don't understand how the body is supposed to function or what certain symptoms are trying to communicate, we risk making decisions that could have serious short- and long-term consequences for our kids.

No one likes to hear this, but it's the truth. And it's a truth that needs to be understood if we want to make better choices for our children.

A Parent's Role

So, what does it mean to have Mental Acuity as a parent?

First, it's having a clear perspective on how your child's body is supposed to work and develop. It's about understanding the design and function of their body so you can assess what's going on accurately, without being misled by surface-level symptoms.

Second, it's about removing the masks that many medical interventions create. Medications and quick fixes often cover up the real issues your child is experiencing. Having Mental Acuity means looking beyond those masks and getting an honest assessment of your child's current health state and understanding what is really happening at its root.

Finally, it's about creating a game plan. Once you understand what's happening, you can start taking actionable steps to help your child move from their current health condition towards restored health and healthy neurodevelopment. This is especially important if your child has been struggling for a long time.

It's not enough to just know what's wrong. You need the wisdom to navigate your child's health challenges with a long-term perspective.

Knowledge vs. Wisdom

A patient of mine once illustrated this beautifully. He was a farmer, and he loved to share stories and his own brand of farmer wisdom. One day he walked into my office and said, "Doc, do you know the difference between knowledge and wisdom?"

I smiled and replied, "Sure I do, but I'd love to hear what you have to say."

He said, "Knowledge is knowing that a tomato is a fruit. Wisdom is knowing not to put a tomato in a fruit salad."

It's a simple but profound distinction. Knowledge is about facts. Wisdom is about application.

As parents, we don't just need to know the facts about our children's health—what a diagnosis is called or what medication can make a symptom disappear. We need the wisdom to understand what those symptoms mean, where they're coming from, and how to address the root cause.

That's the kind of wisdom that can make a lasting difference in your child's life. It's the difference between masking a problem and solving it. Between keeping your child stuck and helping them thrive.

Mental Acuity is foundational to being able to both understand and steward the other five pillars of health well. Without a right perspective on how the body works and what symptoms truly mean, it becomes much harder to make sound decisions for your child. If we don't approach health with clarity and wisdom, our decision-making becomes compromised, affecting not just this moment, but the long-term health and development of our children.

Chapter 4

Emotional Fortitude

Big Emotions for Small People

Dr. Chris

Growing up, did you have a sibling who just loved to scare you? You know the type. They'd sit behind a door, turn off all the lights, and wait until you walked into a room completely unsuspecting. They knew exactly how to get under your skin after years of testing your vulnerabilities, and they'd plan the perfect moment to strike.

Picture it: You walk into a dark room, mind completely elsewhere. You flip on the light, and suddenly—**BAM!**—your sibling leaps out with a yell, scaring you out of your skin. In that moment, everything changes. Your heart races, your body tenses, and your brain goes into overdrive. You're no longer thinking about what's for dinner or your homework—now, you're in survival mode.

Your body takes over completely. You might jump and scream, stumble backward, or freeze with weak knees. Or maybe you go on the offensive and lunge right at them, throwing a punch or a shove. After all, they deserve it—they are your sibling and they scared you.

This reaction is called the fight-or-flight response, and it's your brain's way of protecting you in moments of perceived danger. It's an essential survival mechanism, designed to help us respond quickly to threats. Without it, our ancestors wouldn't have lasted very long in a world full of predators and dangers.

But here's the thing: the fight-or-flight response is fantastic for short-term, immediate threats. When your life is on the line, it sharpens your focus, quickens your reflexes, and pumps adrenaline into your system to make you stronger and faster. Your heart races, blood flow increases to your muscles, and your body is primed for action. These physical changes get you ready to either fight or run away from the threatening situation.

At the same time, however, your body temporarily shuts down "non-essential" functions. Digestion? On hold. Bathroom breaks? Forget it. Clear thinking? Not a priority—because, let's face it, you don't need to be solving algebra equations in the middle of a bear fight. In these moments, your brain is wired to prioritize survival, not long division.

Emotions and the Body

Ultimately the fight-or-flight response is governed by emotions, and the number one emotional trigger of the fight-or-flight response is fear. Fear arises when we believe our life might be in danger. This response is unconscious and often feels completely outside of our control, as do the physical changes that come with it.

In contrast, when a person experiences a sense of safety and security, the body shifts toward the parasympathetic state—the rest-and-digest mode. In this state, the muscles relax, the heart rate slows, and the mind becomes clearer. But more importantly, this is the state in which the body heals most effectively. The immune system operates at its highest capacity, energy is used more efficiently, and healthy reserves are built up. It is in this mode that food is digested, cells are repaired, and the body grows at its best pace. For children, remaining in this parasympathetic state the majority of the time is essential, because it is also where neurodevelopment thrives. It is where the brain is cleansed, new synaptic connections are strengthened, and long-term learning is optimized.

Fear pulls the body into stress and sympathetic tone, where anxiety and stress rise, sleep is disrupted, energy is drained, immunity is weakened, and both growth and repair slow down. Safety pushes the body back into regulation, where strength, health, and resilience are built. These are involuntary responses—an outward display of the inward emotional state.

This direct connection between the emotional state of the brain and the physical state of the body is constant, and the body always reflects the brain's condition. Growth, development, and repair depend on the parasympathetic state. When the nervous system is stuck in sympathetic tone, those critical processes are stunted. This is why a child's sense of safety is so crucial. Safety keeps the nervous system in parasympathetic tone, giving the body the best chance to grow, repair, and develop.

Balancing Safety and Guidance

Younger children need the safety of their parents. They are not equipped to handle adult-level stresses, responsibilities, or fears. While they can manage age-appropriate challenges, their sensitivity to emotional states means that even small emotions can feel massive inside their tiny bodies. A safe and solid connection with mom and dad creates the environment needed to sort these big emotions out.

Children also need parents who carefully guide, direct, and strengthen them over time so they can learn to handle increasing amounts of stress. The goal isn't to shield them from all challenges but to help them develop the resilience needed to face life's difficulties head-on.

This is why helicopter parenting often draws criticism. These parents hover over their children and shield them from adversity. They may even complete tasks on their behalf—tasks that were meant to build independence and skill. While this may feel merciful in the moment, in the long term it creates children who lack resilience and struggle to handle the inevitable challenges of life.

On the other extreme, neglectful parenting is equally damaging. Neglectful parents expose children to prolonged emotional strain or may even be the cause of that strain through inconsistent and hypocritical standards, routines, or habits. This level of stress overwhelms a child's ability to cope, trapping them in a chronic fight-or-flight response.

Adults with strong Emotional Fortitude often had parents who struck this balance well. They were protected from extreme harm but were still allowed to experience difficulties that helped them grow. The result is resilience—the strength to endure life's hardships without being overwhelmed by them.

Building Resilience

Emotional Fortitude is the ability to build resilience over time—the capacity to endure stressful, challenging, or even dangerous situations while keeping the body in a calm and regulated state. A healthy person can handle life's difficulties without being overwhelmed. They can also experience a full range of emotions in a healthy way.

For children, this growth happens in small steps. A child might cry when upset, and with comfort, return quickly to play. Or they may be startled, briefly go into fight-or-flight, but then calm down with reassurance and a hug. Each time they cycle through stress and return to safety, they practice resilience. Over years, these small steps accumulate into a strong capacity for handling life's harder challenges.

Ultimately, healthy parenting means allowing children to become resilient people. Resilient people can stay in a parasympathetic state even when life feels difficult, uncertain, or even threatening. But when safety or guidance is compromised and serious chronic stress persists—like when children live in environments where they feel unsafe or stressed regularly—the body remains in a prolonged state of stress. And that is where the harm begins.

Prolonged stress erodes the body over time. The brain's cognitive function slows, the heart rate stays elevated, blood pressure remains high, and hormonal imbalances worsen. Sleep becomes compromised, posture tightens unnaturally, and a host of other symptoms can appear. Children stuck in this cycle often experience physical and emotional challenges that affect their ability to grow and thrive.

The key to healthy neurodevelopment through every stage of childhood is balance. Children must face challenges to grow stronger and build Emotional Fortitude. At the same time, they need protection from extremes so that their bodies and minds can recover along the way. This balance of challenge and rest is what allows a child to thrive.

Chapter 5

Chemical Purity

A Clean Body Is a Healthy Body

Dr. Chris

I once had a family under my care who had two young boys. They were healthy—full of life and energy. Both of them had been adopted, and their parents were some of the most caring, committed people I've ever met. After a few years, the family adopted a third boy. This time, however, the situation was very different.

The newest member of their family had spent his entire time in utero exposed to heroin. His biological mother, struggling with addiction, had used the drug throughout her pregnancy. By the time the adoption went through, and the little boy came home, he was in dire shape.

Within a couple of weeks of his arrival, the family brought him in to see me. From the moment I met him, I could see just how difficult his journey had been. He was one of the most underdeveloped children I had ever seen.

His muscles were barely formed, his small body was fragile, and his eyes were sunken deep into his skull. He was about half the size he should have been for his age. He felt so frail that I was almost afraid to do much with him at all.

But this family came in with a clear sense of purpose. They knew the challenges ahead and were unwavering in their resolve to help this little boy heal.

Both parents had personally experienced tremendous health improvements through the Upper Cervical Care we provided. They had seen amazing changes in their older boys, too. They knew the importance of ensuring the nervous system was functioning correctly, but they also understood that there are other functions of the body that are critical to manage.

This family was incredibly intentional about their health. They ate well, avoided medications whenever possible, and steered clear of anything with unnecessary chemicals. But their new son hadn't been given that chance. From conception, his tiny body had been bombarded with heroin and malnourished due to his mother's neglect.

Over the next year, I watched as they began the long process of detoxifying his body. They worked diligently to help him eliminate the heroin that had been coursing through his veins and lodging in the cells of his body. It wasn't easy.

But they never let up. They surrounded him with love, nourished him with real, whole foods, and stewarded his health with patience and care. Slowly but surely, his tiny body began to heal.

Over the next couple of years, his development sped up. He began to gain muscle, play hard with his brothers, and laugh like any other child his age. By the time he was about four years old, you wouldn't have noticed a difference between him and any other child on the playground.

His body became chemically pure, and as a result, his health completely transformed. For this little boy, the number one problem affecting his body and brain was chemical toxicity.

The Importance of Chemical Purity

Any time a child is exposed to chemical toxins, it has the potential to interfere with their body's natural functions. To put it simply, toxins are substances the body cannot metabolize. Unlike nutrients (which are the building blocks and fuel for the body), toxins have no role in providing energy or creating new cells. They are foreign substances that the body cannot use productively. They are powerful—but ultimately detrimental.

In a perfect world, the only substances entering the body would be those that can be metabolized—either used as fuel or serving as building blocks for the body's structure. Anything outside of these two categories can be considered a toxin.

Toxins come in many forms. The most obvious ones are household chemicals, such as cleaning products or laundry detergents. Others include environmental toxins like carbon monoxide or lead-contaminated water. However, toxins can also come from less obvious sources, such as pharmaceutical drugs, over-the-counter medications, vaccines, and other injectables. Even the food we eat has become increasingly toxic over time, thanks to the heavy use of pesticides, preservatives, and additives.

While we won't dive into the specifics of which substances are toxic in this book, the principle is simple: when a body accumulates toxins, it cannot function correctly. Put simply, you cannot be toxic and healthy at the same time.

Ironically, many of the things we turn to when we're sick—such as medications and vaccines—contribute to the accumulation of toxins in our bodies. In an effort to manage symptoms or prevent future infections, we often compromise Chemical Purity, a key pillar of health. We trade short-term comfort or perceived protection for long-term harm.

Prioritizing Chemical Purity

To maximize health, we must prioritize Chemical Purity. This means:

- Cleaning up our food sources to avoid toxic additives.
- Limiting exposure to environmental toxins such as cleaning supplies, air pollutants, and water contaminants.

- Reducing or eliminating the introduction of medications, synthesized chemicals, and vaccines into the body. (For more information on vaccine safety and informed consent, go to Appendix C)

When we succeed in maintaining Chemical Purity, the only substances left in the body are those it can use to function optimally. The body becomes a reflection of the quality of the materials it's given. The better the quality, the better the result.

A Chemically Pure Brain

Certain toxins have an even more dangerous characteristic: the ability to cross the blood-brain barrier. This protective layer normally shields the brain and central nervous system from harmful substances. However, some toxins, especially heavy metals, can bypass this barrier and directly impact the brain's function and development.

When toxins infiltrate the central nervous system, they disrupt neural pathways, interfering with the brain's ability to function and develop normally. This can have a profound effect on a child's neurodevelopment. In severe cases, such as heavy metal toxicity, this interference can lead to significant delays in development.

The good news is that tremendous progress can often be made by addressing chemical toxicity. Reducing a child's exposure to harmful substances and using appropriate detoxification methods can restore the brain's function and support healthy development.

The young boy in the earlier story is a perfect example. Although he entered the world with heroin coursing through his system, he was removed from the toxic environment that would have continued to poison him. Instead, he was placed in a clean, nurturing environment where he could detoxify and heal. By the time he reached four years old, his development had normalized to the point where no one would suspect he had such a difficult start.

Not all children are so fortunate. Many are born into toxic environments and remain there, exposed to harmful substances throughout their formative years. These children often face significant and ongoing neurodevelopmental challenges.

For parents, this is a call to action. Protecting your child from chemical toxins is critical for their physical health and even more so for their neurodevelopment. A chemically pure brain is essential for proper growth, learning, and thriving at every stage of life. By prioritizing Chemical Purity, you give your child the best chance for optimal brain development and overall health.

Chapter 6

Nutritional Saturation

Maximum Fuel For Maximum Function

Dr. Chris

As a doctor, I've had countless conversations with parents about their children's nutrition. Over the years, I've seen families of all kinds and children with a wide variety of conditions. Most of the parents I work with are intentional about their children's health. They tend to be naturally minded and strive to nourish their kids well. They prioritize home-cooked meals and aim to avoid toxins, pesticides, and hormones in their food.

Occasionally, I meet parents who don't know where to start. They've never considered changing their child's diet and feel overwhelmed by the idea. Outside the clinical setting, I've also encountered parents who lean on convenience—opting for fast food or snacks like Cheerios to get through the day. For many, financial limitations play a significant role. High-quality food costs more and takes more effort to source and prepare.

We could spend hours discussing how to transition from unhealthy eating habits to healthier ones, how to identify high-quality foods, and how to recognize the specific dangers of low-quality options. But this chapter isn't about creating a checklist of foods to eat or avoid. Instead, it focuses on the principle of Nutritional Saturation: providing the maximum amount of essential nutrients to the body at a cellular level to fuel optimal growth and function.

The Purpose of Nutrition

At its core, nutrition serves two essential purposes:
1. **Fuel**: Providing the energy needed to keep the body running.
2. **Building Blocks**: Supplying the materials required to repair, grow, and maintain the body.

To understand this, let's start with an example: building a car. Imagine you're working on an assembly line. To build a functioning car, you need specific materials—cloth for seats, rubber for tires, metal for the engine, and silicone for computer components. These raw materials must be processed and formed into their respective parts, which are then assembled into a finished vehicle.

If you don't supply the rubber for the tires or the metal for the engine, what happens? The car will be incomplete. The car won't drive. A design only works if the right materials are provided and the parts are put together correctly.

The human body works the same way. It requires raw materials—nutrients like vitamins, minerals, carbohydrates, proteins, and fats—to build its structure and maintain its function. Through digestion, the body breaks down food into these raw materials, repurposes them, and assembles them into muscles, bones, cells, and organs.

Now, let's take the example one step further. Imagine you've provided all the necessary materials to build the car, but there's no fuel in the tank. Even with a flawless design and complete assembly, the car won't run. Similarly, even if children consume enough nutrients to build their bodies, they still need fuel—energy from carbohydrates and fats—to keep those bodies functioning. Without sufficient fuel, a child's body will become sluggish, their brain will struggle to process information, and they'll lack the energy needed to thrive.

Here's another example: building a skyscraper. A skyscraper must support an incredible amount of weight pressing down on its frame and foundation. That's why these buildings require deep, stable foundations and materials with high structural integrity, such as steel I-beams.

Now imagine trying to build the same skyscraper with Tinker Toys. While you could connect the pieces and mimic the structure, the Tinker Toys would collapse under the weight. Similarly, cheap, low-quality food might provide some level of sustenance, but it lacks the "structural integrity" needed to build a strong, resilient body.

Children need high-quality nutrients to grow properly—just as a skyscraper needs I-beams, not Tinker Toys. By prioritizing nutrient-dense, high-quality foods that the body can absorb and use effectively, parents provide their children with the best materials to grow and thrive.

Why Kids Eat A Lot

Children's nutritional needs differ significantly from those of adults. While adults primarily use nutrients for maintenance, children need them for growth and adaptation. Their bodies are constantly building bones, muscles, neural connections, and more—all at an extraordinary pace.

This rapid growth explains why children always seem hungry. Their bodies are burning through energy and nutrients, not just to sustain daily activity, but to fuel the biological processes that drive development. Proportionate to their size, children need far more nutrients than adults. They require both the right quantity and the right quality of nutrients to meet their unique needs.

The Keystone of Nutritional Saturation: Absorption

Eating nutrient-dense foods is only part of the equation. True Nutritional Saturation depends on the body's ability to digest and absorb those nutrients effectively.

No matter how high-quality a child's diet is, if their digestive system isn't functioning properly, their body won't receive the nutrients it needs. Proper gut health is critical because it ensures that food is broken down, nutrients are absorbed into the bloodstream, and those nutrients are delivered to the cells and systems that require them for growth and repair.

In short, full Nutritional Saturation happens only when:

1. Food is digested completely.
2. Nutrients are absorbed efficiently.
3. Nutrients are delivered to the cells and systems that need them.

By focusing on high-quality nutrients, proper digestion, and efficient absorption, parents can provide their children with the foundation they need to thrive.

Remember our example of building a skyscraper: the integrity of the structure depends on the quality of the materials and the strength of the foundation. With the right fuel and building blocks, children can grow strong, resilient, and ready to face the challenges of life.

Chapter 7

Structural Stability

Physical Milestones for a Strong Adulthood

Dr. Chris

I had a young boy under my care for many years, starting when he was just three years old. He was incredibly athletic, always running, climbing, and playing with boundless energy. Over time, his visits became less frequent as his family's schedule grew busier. Then, one day, we received a call from his mother. She sounded alarmed, saying her son needed to come in urgently because his neck wasn't right after an incident in school.

When they arrived, it was immediately clear how serious the situation was. His head was tilted sharply to the side—nearly 90 degrees —with his ear almost touching his shoulder. He couldn't move it at all. His face revealed intense pain, and his entire body leaned awkwardly in an attempt to ease the tension running through his frame.

Naturally, I asked what had happened.

He said, "I was playing football."

"Did you get tackled?" I asked.

"No," he replied, looking sheepish.

"Then what happened?"

"I got hit in the head with the football."

His mother looked both frustrated and concerned. At just six years old, it was clearly an accident, and I reassured them we'd get to the bottom of it.

A quick physical examination confirmed that his neck was completely locked in place. Suspecting a severe muscle spasm or misalignment, we took X-rays—his first ever. The X-rays revealed a significant misalignment in his upper neck, which had triggered what was very obviously torticollis (where the neck muscles contract involuntarily twisting the head to one side). But this was not something he had to simply live with.

We knew what caused it, and after analyzing the X-rays, I knew exactly what to do to fix it. I used our sound wave adjusting instrument to correct the alignment of his atlas bone. It was a gentle but precise correction.

After the adjustment, I had him stay on the table for a few minutes, even though his neck was still tender. When he sat up, his head was already 45 degrees straighter. It wasn't perfect yet, but the progress was remarkable for just one adjustment.

By the next day, his head tilt had reduced to about 10 degrees, and his muscles were much more balanced. After one more adjustment, his neck was completely restored, and within a few days, it was as if the torticollis had never happened.

This young boy was fortunate—he had incredible Structural Stability to begin with because of his athleticism. But one incident disrupted that stability, causing pain, muscle tension, and nerve interference. Restoring his structural alignment was key to helping his body heal and return to its normal function.

The Three Components of Structural Stability

Structural Stability is built on three essential components:

1. **Structural Development**: The body's natural design and growth from conception.
2. **Training and Strengthening**: Building strength and resilience through proper use and activity.

3. **Alignment and Function**: Maintaining proper alignment and motion of the joints to ensure optimal performance and injury prevention.

Let's explore each of these in more detail.

1. Structural Development

The DNA we inherit from our parents serves as the blueprint for our design. This genetic code determines everything from the symmetry of our faces to the strength of our bones and muscles. Under ideal conditions—where the body receives the right nutrients, remains toxin-free, and receives clear nerve signals—this blueprint guides the development of a strong, functional structure.

It's important to recognize that the way the body develops structurally has a direct influence on how well it functions. For example, if a child's spine grows with poor alignment, the pressure can disrupt nerve signals and interfere with normal body processes. Structure sets the stage for how the body operates.

At the same time, function also shapes structure. The signals that control posture influence how straight we stand, and the ways we use our bodies—through activity, movement, or repetitive stress—affect how our bones, joints, and muscles grow. A child who stays active will build strength and stability, while inactivity gradually weakens the body. And once the body weakens, it becomes harder to stay active, creating a cycle that erodes both structure and function.

This relationship is best understood as a feedback loop: good structure supports good function, and proper function maintains strong structure. When this loop is well maintained, everything rises together. When it is neglected, both structure and function decline together. Disruptions to this loop—whether from poor nutrition, toxic exposures, or lack of physical activity—undermine the body's design and resilience. That is why providing children with the right building blocks, such as nutrient-dense food, healthy movement, and clear nerve signals, is so critical to ensuring strong structural development and long-term health.

2. Training and Strengthening

Physical activity does much more than simply burn energy or keep children busy—it plays a critical role in strengthening the body's structure and enhancing its resilience. Regular movement builds muscle, increases bone density, and reinforces ligaments and tendons, all of which contribute to overall stability and function.

As physical demands increase, the body adapts to meet them. Repetitive stress from activity stimulates bone growth, making it denser and more durable, while ligaments and tendons become stronger and more elastic. Even the circulatory system responds, improving blood flow to deliver oxygen and nutrients more efficiently to working tissues. These adaptations not only enhance physical performance but also create a foundation of structural integrity that supports long-term health and injury prevention.

This process of adaptation extends to the nervous system as well, through a mechanism called neuroplasticity. Neuroplasticity is the ability of the nervous system to adapt and grow in response to use. Just like muscles, nerves increase in size and efficiency the more they are used. The pathways between the brain and body become stronger, faster, and more reliable with repeated use, allowing for improved coordination, reaction time, and overall function.

3. Alignment and Function

Alignment is the final piece of Structural Stability, and it plays a critical role in maintaining optimal function.

The spine, in particular, is a vital structure. It houses the spinal cord and the lower part of the brainstem, which transmit nerve signals between the brain and body. The upper neck, or craniocervical junction, is the most vulnerable area of the spine. Misalignments here can disrupt nerve signals, leading to widespread dysfunction in the body.

For example, when the young football player developed torticollis, the misalignment in his neck caused severe muscle tension and nerve interference. Restoring his alignment allowed his muscles to relax and his nerves to function properly again, resolving the issue quickly.

Alignment and function are interconnected. A well-aligned body is less likely to sustain injuries, while a poorly aligned body is more prone to breakdowns that impair function.

Stable Foundations

Structural Stability is a cornerstone of lifelong health. It begins with proper structural development, continues with training and strengthening, and relies on maintaining alignment for optimal function. Children who develop strong, resilient structures and maintain alignment through regular activity and care are less likely to experience injuries or long-term dysfunction.

When structures are weak or misaligned, the body is forced to compensate, often creating strain and dysfunction that ripple through every system. Ensuring stability isn't only about avoiding injuries—it's about giving the body the foundation it needs to grow, adapt, and thrive.

In the next chapter, we'll explore the connection between Structural Stability and Neurological Clarity, the most essential pillar of health.

Chapter 8

Neurological Clarity

Bridging the Systems of the Body Together

Dr. Chris

Early in my career, I had a 16-year-old boy brought into the clinic by his mother. He was an exceptional cross-country runner, known for his speed and ability to win races consistently. But recently, something had changed. His mother explained that for the last few months, during his races, he would develop an asthma attack about three miles in. It happened suddenly and without fail, forcing him to stop running altogether during the race.

This boy was a well-trained athlete. He had been running competitively for years, maintained a healthy lifestyle, and took care of all the essential elements of his health. Yet his asthma attacks had no clear explanation that they could figure out.. His primary doctor had ruled out allergies, and they didn't know where else to turn. They had heard we had helped others with asthma and decided to give our care a try.

I was intrigued. Most cases of asthma I'd seen were triggered by environmental or chemical factors, but this was different. The fact that he could run full speed for miles before the attack suggested something deeper was at play.

After collecting more details, we performed a thorough physical exam and took X-rays. The analysis revealed a misalignment in his upper neck that was directly affecting his brainstem function. This misalignment was compromising the clarity of nerve signals between his brain and body. While I couldn't explain why the symptoms appeared specifically at three miles, it was clear his nervous system was not operating at its full potential.

In this case I also used the Advanced Orthogonal technique, which is the sound wave adjustment I mentioned earlier. After the adjustment, I explained the importance of rest to allow his body to adapt to the restored nerve signals. I advised him to avoid physical activity for a few days and scheduled a follow-up appointment.

When he returned, I asked if he had followed my advice. He hesitated, then admitted he had raced that very same day. I could feel the disappointment on my face, but before I could say anything, he added, "I got first place. And I didn't have any asthma attacks."

I was stunned.

His mother, smiling ear to ear, confirmed it. "He ran faster than he's ever run before," she said.

In just a few hours, his body had adapted to the restored alignment, and the improvement in his athletic performance was undeniable. His lung function was completely normalized, and the asthma symptoms were gone. Over the following weeks, we worked to ensure his neck stayed in alignment long-term. As his body stabilized, his performance continued to improve. The clarity of the nerve signals between his brain and body optimized his athletic ability, and he went on to achieve new personal bests in his races.

This is a perfect example of the principle of Neurological Clarity.

The Bridge That Ties the Body Together

Neurological Clarity is the foundation that allows the brain and body to function in harmony. The brain is the command center of the body, coordinating and controlling every function. For this to happen effectively, the brain needs clear information from the body and must send clear signals back to direct the body's actions. This acts as a continuous feedback loop where the body continuously communicates with the brain and the brain continuously responds according to those signals and the body's needs. This communication loop is essential for health and performance.

When this loop is disrupted, the body cannot function at its full potential. Signals from the body to the brain may be incomplete or distorted, leaving the brain unaware of what's happening. Conversely, signals from the brain to the body may be weak or incorrect, leading to dysfunction in critical processes.

This feedback loop is what makes Neurological Clarity so important. Without it, the other pillars of health cannot function optimally:

- **Mental Acuity**: The brain relies on clear signals to process information, focus, and make decisions. Neurological Clarity enhances these cognitive functions.

- **Emotional Fortitude**: Emotional regulation depends on the limbic system, which processes and balances emotional responses. Clear communication between the brain and body ensures healthy emotional processing and resilience.

- **Chemical Purity**: The body's detoxification systems are directed by the brain. Clear signals are necessary to identify toxins, coordinate their removal, and maintain overall chemical balance.

- **Nutritional Saturation**: While nutrients fuel and build the nervous system, the brain also governs digestion, absorption, and nutrient delivery. Neurological Clarity ensures these processes work seamlessly.

- **Structural Stability**: The brain directs the growth, repair, and alignment of the body's framework. Without clear nerve signals, even a well-built structure can become compromised.

Neurological Clarity is the key that ties all these pillars together. It ensures that the systems of the body can communicate and work as one cohesive unit.

Barriers to Neurological Clarity

Several factors can interfere with nerve signaling, disrupting Neurological Clarity and preventing the body from functioning at its full potential. One of the most significant barriers is structural misalignment, particularly in the craniocervical junction—the upper neck region where the brainstem transitions into the spinal cord. This area is the most sensitive and vulnerable joint structure in the spine, and when misaligned, it can directly interfere with nerve communication. While misalignments can occur in other parts of the spine, none have the same neurological impact as those in the craniocervical junction. A disruption here can cause global dysfunction, affecting nearly every system in the body.

Beyond structural issues, chemical toxicity presents another challenge. Toxins that accumulate in the body—whether from food, environmental exposure, or medical interventions—can weaken or distort nerve signals. Chemical interference in the synaptic connections between the nerves can alter how nerves communicate, leading to erratic or diminished signals that compromise clarity. This toxicity can slow down or impair crucial processes, making it harder for the nervous system to regulate bodily functions efficiently.

In addition to chemical interference, nutritional depletion plays a crucial role in diminishing Neurological Clarity. The nervous system requires essential nutrients to maintain the strength and efficiency of nerve signaling. When the body lacks these critical building blocks, the signals traveling between the brain and body can weaken, slowing down communication and reducing overall function. Without proper nutrition, the nervous system struggles to maintain homeostasis, impacting everything from cognitive performance to immune regulation.

Lastly, prolonged stress is a major factor that prevents the nervous system from functioning optimally. A child growing up in an environment filled with inconsistency, lack of structure, or frequent emotional upheaval will struggle to develop proper neurological patterns. Stress keeps the nervous system in a heightened state of fight-or-flight, making it difficult to establish healthy habits, regulate emotions, or adapt to challenges. In contrast, a stable environment—one with routine, peace, and supportive relationships—allows the brain to develop strong, reliable pathways that support emotional and mental resilience.

Each of these barriers—structural misalignment, chemical toxicity, nutritional depletion, and chronic stress—creates interference in the body's ability to send and receive clear signals. Addressing these barriers is essential to restoring Neurological Clarity and ensuring that the brain and body can function in harmony.

Why Neurological Clarity Matters

Neurological Clarity is the bridge that allows the systems of the body to function in harmony. It's not just one of the Six Pillars of Health—it's the pillar that integrates and supports all the others. Without it, even the best efforts in the categories Mental Acuity, Emotional Fortitude, Chemical Purity, Nutritional Saturation, and Structural Stability will fall short.

It's like the cables of a suspension bridge, holding everything together and ensuring stability. When nerve signals are clear, the body can adapt, repair, and thrive. But when these signals are compromised, the entire system is at risk.

Neurological Clarity is not just about optimizing one area of health—it's about ensuring the body can function as a cohesive whole. By addressing structural misalignments, reducing toxicity, creating a peaceful environment, and supporting the nervous system with proper nutrition, parents can optimize their child's brain-body communication and overall health.

From Principles to Practice: A Journey Through Neurodevelopment

Hopefully you now have a foundational understanding of what supports healthy neurodevelopment. These principles are the bedrock upon which a child's brain, body, and nervous system are built. But understanding the principles is just the beginning. To truly grasp how to support your child's growth, we need to explore how these pillars come to life across the stages of development.

In the next few chapters, Dr. Ethan Surprenant will guide you through the stages of neurodevelopment, highlighting the critical milestones, influences, and potential challenges that shape your child's brain and body from conception to adulthood. Stage by stage, he will show you the factors that nurture thriving neurodevelopment and the obstacles that can derail it.

This book isn't intended to be an exhaustive encyclopedia covering every nutritional nuance or rare genetic condition. Instead, think of it as a practical guide—one that helps you recognize the most important influences on your child's brain and nervous system development. Whether you're starting from the very beginning or making changes later in your child's journey, the goal is to help you stay on track or get back on track as early as possible. Along the way, you'll gain tools to recognize signs of healthy progress and, just as importantly, notice when something may be veering off course.

The journey of neurodevelopment begins long before birth. During pregnancy, the baby's developing nervous system is highly influenced by the mother's environment, nutrition, stress levels, and chemical exposures. Every aspect of a mother's well-being—from the foods she eats to the toxins she avoids—affects how the baby's brain and body develop. This early stage is critical for laying the groundwork for proper neural connectivity, reflex development, and immune function.

Birth is a highly complex process that plays a significant role in shaping a baby's nervous system. The natural pressures of labor on the baby help clear the lungs, activate the baby's proprioceptive system, and trigger essential reflexes that prepare them for life outside the womb. However, complications during delivery—such as prolonged labor, medical interventions, or birth trauma—can interfere with these processes and create structural or neurological challenges that may persist beyond birth.

During infancy, a baby's nervous system is primarily focused on four essential functions: eating, sleeping, pooping, and moving. These foundational processes set the stage for neurological organization, physical development, and immune health. When any of these functions are disrupted—such as difficulty latching, frequent colic, irregular digestion, or poor sleep patterns—it can be an early sign of underlying nervous system dysfunction.

During toddlerhood, children engage in an explosion of learning through repetition, movement, exploration, and trial-and-error experiences. Every new action—whether attempting a first word, stacking blocks, climbing onto furniture, or running across the room—lays the groundwork for the development of neural pathways. This stage is when neuroplasticity is at its peak, meaning the brain rapidly strengthens and refines the connections that will later support more advanced functions like speech, problem-solving, and coordination. A toddler's ability to explore freely and engage in repeated physical and cognitive tasks is essential for optimizing brain development during this phase.

As children move into early childhood, many of them begin to show more pronounced signs of either strong neurodevelopment or developmental delays. This stage is often marked by fatigue and frustration, especially if a child has been operating under neurological stress since infancy. Much of this stress is wrapped up in the limbic system, the emotional center of the brain responsible for processing emotions, managing stress, and regulating behavioral responses. When the limbic system is overwhelmed—whether due to unresolved structural issues, persistent stress, or environmental toxins—children may struggle with emotional regulation, social interactions, and cognitive processing.

By the time children reach the grade school years, they face new challenges tied to increased independence and academic expectations. This period is characterized by greater social interaction, structured learning environments, and the early development of executive functioning skills. While these experiences provide critical neurostimulation, they can also magnify existing neurological challenges if earlier developmental issues were left unaddressed. Struggles with focus, sensory processing, and emotional regulation often become more evident during this stage.

Adolescence introduces a powerful new influence: hormonal changes. These changes act as amplifiers, intensifying whatever state the body is already in. If the nervous system is functioning optimally, hormones can enhance resilience, strength, and cognitive ability. However, if underlying dysfunctions have persisted through childhood, adolescence can magnify issues like anxiety, depression, chronic fatigue, and emotional instability.

Adulthood is where the sum total of childhood experiences—both positive and negative—fully materialize. If health was stewarded well in the early years, adulthood is typically marked by strength, resilience, and adaptability. However, unresolved neurological dysfunctions from childhood often carry over, leading to chronic stress, metabolic issues, and other long-term health problems. While neurodevelopment slows significantly in adulthood, the brain still retains some degree of plasticity, meaning that it's never too late to correct dysfunctions and optimize health.

Understanding the trajectory of neurodevelopment across these stages equips parents with the tools to recognize when milestones are being missed, when signs of dysfunction arise, and how to act early to correct a child's path. Neurodevelopment is a lifelong journey, but the earlier issues are identified and addressed, the easier it is to restore proper function. With the right knowledge and interventions, parents can help their children build a strong foundation for health, not just during their formative years, but for life.

So, without further ado, let's begin this journey. Dr. Ethan will take it from here, starting with prenatal development.

Chapter 9

Prenatal Development

Building a Foundation for a Lifetime

Dr. Ethan

"*God Gave Us You?* What is this?" I asked, examining the cover of the little board book my wife handed me as I sat down on the couch of our one-room rental house—a converted shed.

"Just read it," she implored.

As I read, daft as I was, I got to the line: 'Mama, where did I come from?' little cub asked...

"Wait, are you pregnant!?" I blurted out, looking up in shock.

"Yes!" she replied, pulling out a test with two little lines, her face bright with excitement. "Are you happy?" she asked hesitantly, her voice tinged with worry that I might be mad or disappointed.

"Of course!" I said, pulling her close. "We're going to have a baby!"

We were excited. And nervous. And scared. And hopeful. *Oh wow. What will our parents say?* I thought. *Can we afford this baby? What's going to happen when we move to start school?*

The difficulties of the previous pregnancy still lingered in our hearts and minds. *No,* I thought to myself, pulling my wife closer. *This one will be different. We will get to meet this little blessing.*

Destined for Life

My wife and I didn't live an unhealthy life, or so we thought. But a lost baby and a renewed second chance at becoming parents awakened a conscious and focused drive to ensure this baby's environment (mama's womb) was the perfect setting to grant our first child a stable foundation for a life of health.

From the moment of conception, the intricate process of the baby's physical and neural development begins, influenced by the Six Pillars of Health: Mental Acuity, Emotional Fortitude, Chemical Purity, Nutritional Saturation, Structural Stability, and Neurological Clarity. These pillars work in harmony to shape the development of a child in the womb, establishing the foundation for lifelong health and resilience.

A baby's body is designed to prioritize its own development. At the same time, the mother's body has to juggle both her and the baby's needs simultaneously. The baby will draw on every available resource to grow, but the quality of those resources is entirely dependent on the mother's surroundings and choices. Understanding how each pillar influences prenatal development provides a framework for supporting both mother and baby during this critical time.

In this chapter, we'll explore how the Six Pillars of Health directly impact a child's development in the prenatal phase. However, it's important to note that these pillars don't stop being essential after birth. In fact, they remain critical throughout childhood and into adulthood. What changes is the complexity of the challenges that arise when these pillars are not properly stewarded. Over time, unresolved issues can grow in magnitude, but the foundational principles remain the same.

Inside the womb, the mother serves as the direct provider of these Six Pillars. To affect the baby directly, it is the mother who must make the changes. Once the baby is born, the child gradually takes on more responsibility for maintaining these elements of health until reaching full independence as an adult, where all the responsibility falls on them. The essential elements needed to thrive remain unchanged, only the method of delivery shifts. Let's begin by exploring how Mental Acuity plays a vital role during this formative period.

Mental Acuity: A Clear Mind for a Healthy Pregnancy

Pregnancy brings with it a whirlwind of changes—physical, emotional, and relational. Navigating these shifts, sifting through medical advice, and managing daily health practices requires clarity. For both mother and baby to thrive, it takes a right understanding of the nature of pregnancy, the importance of the mother's health, the responsibility of the father, and the supportive roles of community and healthcare providers. This is where Mental Acuity comes in. Being mentally acute during pregnancy begins with this understanding: pregnancy is not pathology, and birth is not an inherently traumatic process. Both pregnancy and birth are part of a natural design. When the body is in right order, pregnancy can be a wonderful experience. Even when certain pillars are less than ideal—excessive stress, inadequate nutrition, or limited support—both mother and baby possess an incredible resilience that can allow them to move toward their highest potential for health.

In most cases, pregnancy and human development follows a natural design: the union of male and female leads to fertilization, which initiates the formation of a unique genetic code (DNA). This new genetic blueprint—distinct from both mother and father, yet carrying inherited traits—contains the instructions for development. Those instructions direct the egg to implant to the uterine wall, and guide the complex process of development–cell division, organ system distinction, and neurologic organization. Pregnancy, then, is not a pathology nor birth a traumatic anomaly—it is a deeply rooted, life-giving design.

Yet in today's world, a far more common narrative paints pregnancy and birth in a less than favorable light. Pop culture often portrays it as chaotic and painful—complete with bumbling fathers, irritable and even belligerent mothers, overbearing relatives, and emergency room drama. Hollywood scripts and family horror stories alike often reinforce the idea that labor is something only to be endured with fear, not embraced with excitement. As a result, birth has become something of an emergency to manage, rather than a natural process to support. Many mothers are never told that birth can happen outside of a hospital, let alone that it can be peaceful, instinctive, and even empowering. The prevailing belief is that more doctors, more drugs, and more interventions are the safest—and only—path forward.

To embrace pregnancy and birth as natural, mothers must first recognize that pregnancy itself is a beautifully coordinated, purposeful process. From the moment of conception, a mother's body begins an extraordinary transformation—not by accident, but by design. Every shift in posture, every fluctuation of energy from high to low, every hormonal change, every strange craving has purpose. The mother's body and developing baby are simultaneously preparing for birth. When mothers understand this, they can be empowered to care for their bodies not out of fear, but with confidence.

The journey of pregnancy is ideally not one the mother should have to walk alone—but for many women, that is their reality. Some face pregnancy without the support of a partner, whether because of abandonment, loss, distance, or circumstances outside their control. Others walk through it with a partner who is physically present but emotionally absent. These situations carry unique burdens, and to the mothers who find themselves there: your strength, resilience, and courage matter deeply, and your child's life still has immeasurable worth.

At the same time, it must be said plainly: when a father is present, he carries a responsibility. Pregnancy is not a season for passivity. A father is called to be more than a bystander—he is meant to be a steady, life-giving presence. His role is to help his partner hold fast to truth when the world offers confusion, to encourage her toward healthy choices, and to protect her from voices that undermine the body's design. This is not control—it is covering. A father leads not just by what he says, but by how he lives: modeling health, clarity, and conviction. His consistency and courage help create a foundation of peace for both mother and child. His strength doesn't overpower—it empowers. We won't be covering all of the ways a father can lead and support his growing family in this book, but for more resources on the father's role, see Appendix C.

Mothers and fathers are very capable of raising their children themselves, but greater strength comes from the support of community. It is especially life giving to the parents when that community affirms the goodness of family and the beauty of natural order. Whether through trusted family and friendships, church communities, co-ops, recreational groups, or outreach gatherings, surrounding themselves with like-minded support is essential. These communities help anchor the parents' mindset, protect their health decisions, and remind them that they are not alone in choosing a better way. The old saying rings true, "*It takes a village to raise a child.*" However, that village begins forming long before the child is born.

Part of building that village includes being intentional about who is invited into the most sensitive spaces—especially the realm of healthcare. Parents should select providers that are not only knowledgeable, but also aligned with a view of health that honors natural design and supports the parents' values. Not all advice is created equal. Not every doctor understands the long term consequences of any single decision. Parents must learn to evaluate every suggestion through the lens of what promotes true health for both mother and baby. That means questioning fear-driven interventions, rejecting blanket advice like "don't exercise, only rest" or "you *have* to be induced between 38 and 41 weeks, any longer and it won't be safe" and standing firm when pressured into one-size-fits-all decisions. Whether it's induction timelines, vaccine schedules, or lifestyle choices, parents have the right—and the responsibility—to say no when something contradicts their priorities. Setting boundaries isn't rebellion—it's wisdom. To help you start finding the right providers for your family as well as to help sort through natural means of pregnancy, delivery, and vaccinations, see the resources in Appendix B and C.

For couples who have not yet married or have not yet had children, it's vital to have these conversations early. Understanding foundational principles of health and each other's perspectives before marriage or before children enter the picture lays the groundwork for a united approach. Establishing these shared values ahead of time minimizes conflict and creates a stable environment for future decision-making.

Emotional Fortitude: Resilience Through the Strength of Unity

Because pregnancy is a season of extraordinary demands—physical, emotional, and logistical—resilience in navigating these challenges while maintaining emotional stability for the baby is crucial for a smooth pregnancy. This resilience, or Emotional Fortitude, is both intrinsic and extrinsic, that is, reinforced by the mother's personal understanding (intrinsic) as well as the understanding the father, family, community, and medical team (extrinsic).

The reason that Emotional Fortitude is so critical during pregnancy is because of the profound effects that stress hormones have on a baby's development (remember the parasympathetic and sympathetic discussed in chapter 4). A developing baby gets its first impressions of the outside world through the mother's internal environment, especially through the blood. If the mother has constant stress or consistent fears, then the baby will be exposed to an increase of stress hormones —cortisol, epinephrine, norepinephrine—over a long period of time, causing a detrimental effect on growth and development from a very early point. It is the same as adults. People do not grow or heal well under stress and fear, and babies are no exception.

At its core, it is easier to maintain Emotional Fortitude in the context of love and stability, and there is no stronger foundation for that stability than the covenant of marriage. Babies are biologically designed to grow within the love and security that marriage provides. Marriage is not merely a legal or ceremonial union—it is a commitment of unity that fosters peace, anchors relationships, and establishes an environment where both mother and baby can thrive. When a mother and father are anchored in a covenant of love and mutual responsibility, the relationship is on solid ground, and there is less stress, especially regarding the uncertainties of the future.

As the mother carries the physical burden of pregnancy, the father has a vital role to play in managing, protecting, and providing to reduce her stress. In its most ideal form, this partnership works in harmony, allowing the mother to focus on nurturing the baby while the father takes on practical responsibilities. These include ensuring financial stability, maintaining a peaceful and organized home environment, and advocating for the mother's needs during medical appointments. The less strain the mother experiences, the more peace she can cultivate, which directly benefits the baby's neurodevelopment by reducing unnecessary stress responses.

While personal resilience is essential, Emotional Fortitude is not developed in isolation. It flourishes within the context of a committed relationship and a broader support network. Trusted friendships and family connections can offer practical assistance and emotional encouragement, but it's critical to set boundaries where necessary. As discussed in Mental Acuity, relationships that introduce conflict or undermine the mother's confidence can be detrimental. It is at its root a source of stress. Protecting the peace and stability of the household by maintaining healthy boundaries ensures that the mother can focus on her well-being and the development of her baby.

This is where the broader concept of environment becomes essential. A mother's environment during pregnancy profoundly affects her emotional state and, by extension, the baby's development. Consider this Biblical parable: A seed planted in rocky soil will struggle to grow deep roots. A seed planted on a busy street may be trampled or swept away. A seed planted among weeds will be choked out. But a seed planted in rich, fertile soil will grow deep, unmovable roots and flourish to its fullest potential. Similarly, a mother's peace, stability, and support create the fertile soil in which a baby can grow and develop to their maximum potential. There are carryover effects of the mothers stress that play into the neurodevelopment of the child. The more stress a mother experiences during pregnancy, the more the child has the potential to develop unhealthy neurological patterns that can affect the child later in their neurodevelopment.

Ultimately, Emotional Fortitude is about creating an environment of peace, stability, and unity where both the mother and baby can flourish. Marriage and a strong support system create fertile soil by providing security, love, and a shared sense of purpose. As the father plays a vital role in minimizing stress and offering support, the mother is better able to remain emotionally resilient and focused on nurturing the baby. This lays the groundwork for the baby's lifelong health and emotional regulation.

Chemical Purity: Minimizing Harmful Exposures

The baby's developing systems are exceptionally sensitive to their environment. After fertilization, the baby attaches to the uterine wall and begins to share blood flow with the mother through the placenta.

The placenta serves as the baby's lifeline, acting as both a gateway and a barrier between mother and child. This intricate organ not only delivers oxygen and essential nutrients but also plays a crucial role in protecting the developing baby from harmful substances. The placental barrier is selectively permeable, meaning it allows beneficial molecules —like antibodies that strengthen the baby's immune system—to pass through while blocking many toxins, bacteria, and larger pathogens that could pose a risk. However, this barrier is not infallible. Certain chemicals (alcohol, opioid medications, microplastics), heavy metals (mercury, cadmium), and infections (toxoplasma parasites, rubella, herpes simplex virus, etc.) can still cross into the baby's bloodstream, potentially disrupting neurodevelopment and organ formation. Even the stress hormones discussed in the previous pages can cross this barrier and cause adverse developmental effects. While the placenta provides an incredible level of protection, the quality of what enters the mother's body directly influences what reaches the baby.

In an ideal world, the only substances entering the body would be nutrients that can be metabolized into energy or become building blocks for new cells and structures in the baby's body. However, exposure to harmful chemicals, whether through medications, cleaning products, pesticides, or environmental toxins—can disrupt the intricate processes of neurodevelopment and organ formation. This makes maternal health choices—such as minimizing toxin exposure, switching to more natural cleaning alternatives, consuming clean and nutrient-dense foods, and supporting immune function with good hygiene and adequate vitamins and minerals—critical in safeguarding the baby's development.

Chemical Purity begins even before conception. Both parents can take steps to detoxify their bodies and minimize exposure to harmful substances before pregnancy. During pregnancy, these habits become even more critical. A mother's choices about food quality, cleaning products, and medications directly influence the baby's exposure to potential toxins.

Reducing chemical exposure is not about achieving perfection but about making intentional choices to create the healthiest environment possible. Every effort—no matter how small—makes a meaningful difference in supporting the baby's development and minimizing the risk of disruptions caused by harmful substances.

Nutritional Saturation: Fueling Optimal Development

A mother's body is designed to prioritize the baby's nutritional needs, directing essential nutrients to the baby first. This process is remarkable but places significant demands on the mother, requiring her to consume nutrient-dense foods to support both herself and her baby.

These nutrients serve as the building blocks for the baby's body and brain. For example, omega-3 fatty acids support critical brain development, while calcium and magnesium contribute to the formation of strong bones and muscles. Every nutrient plays a role in ensuring the baby develops a foundation for lifelong health. However, when a mother's diet is lacking in key nutrients or her digestive health is impaired, the baby may experience deficiencies that could lead to developmental challenges.

True Nutritional Saturation for the baby isn't just about eating whole, healthy foods. It is dependent on the mother's ability to absorb and deliver nutrients effectively. If digestion or absorption are compromised, the baby may not receive the full spectrum of essential vitamins, minerals, and macronutrients needed for proper development.

It's important to note that children's nutritional needs far exceed those of adults in proportion to their size. During pregnancy, a baby's rapid growth and development demand high levels of energy and raw materials. The mother's ability to meet these demands is vital, as the baby depends entirely on her for its nutrients. If the mother's body is unable to supply what the baby requires, her own reserves are depleted, potentially leaving her at risk for nutritional deficiencies and other health complications.

Parents, and especially mothers, have a significant responsibility in ensuring Nutritional Saturation during pregnancy. The mother's choices —both in the quality of her food and the health of her digestive tract —determine whether the baby receives the nutrients it needs to thrive. This principle underscores the importance of understanding how nutrition works at a deeper level, particularly in the context of supporting the body's processes for absorption and nutrient delivery.

Although we won't go into detailed dietary recommendations here, resources are available for parents who want to learn more about this topic. For more in-depth understanding, please refer to the resources in Appendix C. The key to understand here is that maximum nourishment for mom during pregnancy provides maximum nourishment for the baby. Hyper-restrictive diets do not help neurodevelopment. They have the potential to stunt growth. So don't be afraid to eat a fair bit more as long as the quality of the food is very high. It's good for the mother and it's good for the baby.

Structural Stability: Building a Strong Foundation

The baby's skeletal system, muscles, and connective tissues develop in a precise sequence, creating the framework for future movement and strength. These structures rely on the mother's ability to provide the necessary building blocks through her nutritional intake, as we just covered. It is also dependent on her capacity to create a structurally sound environment in which the baby can develop.

As a mother progresses through pregnancy, the temptation to remain sedentary increases. Friends, relatives, and well-meaning strangers often say, "Oh sweetie, you should lay down and get some rest." While this advice may come from a place of care, it is a trap. A sedentary mother is more likely to experience birth complications, develop gestational diabetes, or face residual chronic health issues. If excessive maternal rest can lead to such complications, imagine the impact that inactivity has on the baby's development.

A structurally stable mother is one who uses her body the way it was designed. Growing a baby is no small task, and delivering that baby is a marathon, not a sprint. Mothers should view themselves as athletes and train accordingly. Daily activities like walking, pelvic floor therapy, deep core strengthening, and weight training can transform the mother's body into a fortress, ready to birth. Beyond the benefits to mom, exercise during pregnancy has the benefit of increasing the baby's lean muscle mass even while in utero. A baby with well-prepared muscles will have an easier time progressing through developmental milestones.

Within the concept of Structural Stability lies the proper alignment and mobility of the mother's pelvis. This alignment is critical for guiding the baby into the correct head-down position for an optimal birth. Misalignment or immobility in the pelvis or sacrum can interfere with the baby's positioning. How is this? Baby's have unique primitive reflexes that are designed to be used to orient baby into proper position for birth. The reflexes while in utero cue the baby into a head down orientation. Chiropractic care, acupuncture, and other trained prenatal holistic practices can play a pivotal role in releasing tension in the pelvis and round ligaments while aligning the sacrum. This creates an optimal space for the baby to trigger primitive reflexes and move into the proper position, increasing the likelihood of a smooth delivery.

Structural Stability is more than just physical development for the mother—it sets the foundation for the baby's motor milestones, physical resilience, and overall health. A well-supported pregnancy ensures the baby's framework develops as intended, preparing them for life outside the womb.

Neurological Clarity: Wiring the Brain and Body

By the end of the first month, the baby's neural tube—the precursor to the brain and spinal cord—has already formed. From that point forward, neurons grow and connect at an extraordinary rate, creating the framework for all future learning, movement, and cognition. As these sensitive structures develop, the baby's skull and spine also begin to form, providing protection for the brain, spinal cord, and nervous system.

This process is delicate and highly dependent on the mother's well-being. Proper nutrition, reduced toxin exposure, focused physical activity, and minimized stress are essential for ensuring that the nervous system develops with clarity and precision. Any disruption during this critical time can have lasting effects on the baby's ability to process information and interact with their environment.

By midway through the prenatal period, the baby's sensory systems are already connecting to the outside world. Hearing develops around 18 to 20 weeks, allowing the baby to recognize familiar voices in preparation for life outside the womb. Touch and proprioception (body awareness) emerge early, helping the baby interact with its environment within the womb. The reflexes discussed earlier develop later in pregnancy, closer to 30 weeks. These neurologic reactions to physical touch, light, and sound help position the baby for optimal birth.

As the prenatal period nears its end, from roughly 30 to 42 weeks, the baby's nervous system undergoes an extraordinary refinement process. Neural networks strengthen, reflexes become more coordinated, and the brain begins rehearsing patterns it will rely on immediately after birth—breathing rhythms, swallowing, and the regulation of sleep-wake cycles. Neurological Clarity serves as the organizer of the entire developmental process, integrating the other pillars of health—mental, emotional, structural, chemical, and nutritional—into one unified system. For parents, this underscores the importance of ensuring that the mother's nervous system functions with clarity, free of structural misalignments, so brain-to-body communication remains strong and the developing child can enter the world with the most stable foundation possible.

Long-Term Implications

The prenatal period establishes the groundwork for lifelong health. When the Six Pillars of Health are carefully stewarded, the baby has the best chance to thrive. Conversely, disruptions in any of these areas—

such as poor nutrition, excessive stress, or toxin exposure—can lead to lasting challenges in neurodevelopment, motor milestones, and emotional regulation.

Accurately understanding and applying these principles early ensures the baby starts life with a strong foundation, ready to meet developmental milestones and adapt to life outside the womb. A healthy prenatal environment directly influences how the baby transitions into the world and their ability to grow, learn, and flourish.

As the baby completes its prenatal journey, the transition to birth becomes a defining moment. This critical phase activates the baby's neurological, hormonal, and structural systems, setting the stage for life outside the womb. But what happens when this process doesn't go as nature intended?

In the next chapter, we'll uncover how the birth process shapes future neurodevelopment and why its impact can leave lasting ripples, for better or worse.

Chapter 10

The Birth Process

Transitioning to the Outside World

Dr. Ethan

Birth marks one of life's most profound transitions, shifting the baby from the safety of the womb to the complexities of the outside world. This natural process is intricately designed to prepare both mother and baby for this monumental change. While birth introduces significant physical and physiological stress, this stress plays a vital role in activating the baby's neurologic, hormonal, and structural systems—preparing it to breathe, feed, and adapt to life outside the womb.

The prenatal stage establishes the foundation for development, ensuring that by the time labor begins, the baby's major systems are fully formed. Labor and delivery then serve as the initiation point where these systems are tested against the outside world. While labor may feel long and intense for many mothers, it is relatively short compared to nine months of prenatal development and the decades of life that follow. Yet in this critical moment, the way a baby enters the world can have lasting implications for health and neurodevelopment.

Birth as a Natural Process

Just like we mentioned briefly in the previous chapter, the birth process is naturally orchestrated to help the baby transition to life outside the womb. Each element of the process serves a distinct purpose:

- **Neurologic Activation:** The pressure and movement experienced during birth stimulate proprioceptive feedback loops, activating the baby's nervous system and preparing motor and sensory functions.
- **Hormonal Preparation:** Oxytocin released during labor helps the baby connect with the mother, regulate temperature, and adapt to its new environment.
- **Clearing the Lungs:** The compression of the chest during vaginal delivery expels amniotic fluid from the lungs, enabling the baby to take its first breath.

When the birth process unfolds naturally, these stressors work in harmony, allowing the baby to transition smoothly to life outside of the mother's womb. However, when this process is disrupted or bypassed, the consequences can ripple through the baby's development.

A Traumatic Start to Life

"Dad, I've got some news," the doctor said calmly, even amid the stressful situation of marathon labor. "Your baby is stuck. We'll need to perform a cesarean to deliver him."

Hearing the doctor, my (Dr. Ethan's) dad carefully watched the fetal monitoring strip, the signs of his son's distress appearing on the printed lines. After a moment in prayer and a quick confirmation from my mom, my dad gave the go-ahead, "We are good, do what you have to."

As the doctor performed the operation, my dad watched carefully, wanting to be fully attentive for his wife and new baby. Once the doctor pulled me out, he called to my dad, "Are you ready to cut the cord?"

Tentatively stepping below the partition, my dad announced proudly, "It's a boy! Ethan Alexander Surprenant!" He cut the cord, and I was brought next to my mother for the first time. She lovingly caressed my head, whispering softly, "Hey, little buddy. It's good to meet you."

My birth story is not uncommon. According to the CDC, just over 30% of births in the United States are performed via cesarean section. By contrast, the World Health Organization recommends that only 10–15% of births involve C-sections, emphasizing the importance of natural delivery whenever possible. This disparity indicates that modern hospitals are directing mothers toward surgical interventions at more than double the globally recommended rate.

These interventions disrupt the natural processes of birth that are crucial for the baby's neurologic activation, hormonal regulation, and physical stability. They can create a cascade of challenges, including respiratory distress, increased sympathetic overload, and structural strain for both mother and baby.

The Overlooked Factor: Structural Strain

While birth is a natural process, it introduces significant physical forces, particularly on the baby's head, neck, and spine. Ironically, while healthcare providers routinely evaluate the baby's heart, lungs, and reflexes, the structural alignment of the baby's spine—the keystone of neurologic signaling and function—is rarely examined.

The spinal cord serves as the body's primary communication highway, carrying signals between the brain and the body. A baby's ability to breathe, feed, digest, and regulate vital systems relies on clear, uninterrupted nerve signals along this pathway. Physical strain during birth can misalign the baby's spine, disrupting these signals and leading to issues such as feeding difficulties, colic, and sleep disruptions.

In fact, a 2015 study found that 99% of newborns within 72 hours of birth had somatic dysfunction in the skull, upper cervical spine, or sacrum—three critical areas for neurologic function. Yet, structural evaluations are often overlooked, except by chiropractors or specialists trained to assess spinal alignment.

The forces involved in delivery, even under normal circumstances, are substantial. Modern medical interventions amplify these forces:

- **Forceps or Vacuum Extractors:** While these tools assist in delivery, they can exert excessive pressure on the baby's cranial bones and upper cervical spine.
- **Manual Pulling and C-sections:** The force used during these procedures can misalign the baby's delicate skeletal structures.
- **Induced Labor and Epidurals:** Artificially increasing contractions with Pitocin and limiting the mother's ability to respond to labor with an epidural increase the strain on both mother and baby.

While sometimes necessary, these interventions can leave lasting structural challenges, including misalignments that disrupt neurologic signaling and contribute to digestive issues, sleep disturbances, and developmental delays.

Neurodevelopmental Implications

One of the most common early challenges is feeding difficulties, where nerve disruptions in the brainstem interfere with a baby's ability to latch, suck, and swallow effectively. The coordination required for breastfeeding or bottle-feeding depends on coordinated and clear neural pathways between the mouth, throat, and digestive system. If these pathways are compromised due to birth trauma, feeding struggles can arise.

Similarly, digestive challenges like colic, excessive gas, constipation, or reflux—common concerns for many parents—often have a neurological basis. The Vagus nerve (a nerve from the brainstem and running through the upper cervical region) and the sacral plexus (a group of nerves originating from the sacral region) are the main coordinators of the digestive process. When nerve signals between the gut and brainstem are disrupted from spinal misalignment in the cranial bones, upper cervical spine, and sacrum, the digestive system cannot function optimally, resulting in discomfort and irregular bowel movements.

Sleep disruptions can also be linked to structural misalignments introduced during birth. Restorative sleep (covered in depth in the next chapter) requires the body to transition into a parasympathetic state—the nervous system mode responsible for relaxation and recovery. If a baby's nervous system remains in a heightened state of stress due to unresolved birth trauma, sleep may be fragmented, restless, or insufficient, leading to increased fussiness and difficulty when self-soothing.

The effects of these structural disruptions can extend beyond infancy, delaying developmental milestones and creating a cascade of challenges as the child grows. A baby who struggles with feeding or digestion may experience slower weight gain, poor nutrient absorption, and weakened immune function. Sleep disturbances in infancy can set the stage for dysregulated sleep patterns later in childhood, affecting cognitive function and emotional stability. Unresolved structural misalignments may also contribute to motor delays, posture issues, or sensory processing difficulties as the child develops.

Building the skills to limit the need for interventions and structural stressors introduced during birth is essential for establishing a solid foundation for infancy. By supporting the baby's transition to the outside world and addressing these early challenges, parents can set their child on the path to thrive. For detailed steps on a more natural approach to birth check out the resources in Appendix C.

But how do you know if your baby's development is on track? In the next chapter, we'll uncover the four essential jobs of infancy—sleeping, eating, pooping, and moving—and how these seemingly simple tasks reveal the health and balance of your baby's nervous system.

Chapter 11

Infancy

Balance, Growth, and Adaptation

Dr. Ethan

The telephone rang, and after a moment, I heard a mother's voice answer.

"Hello?" she said.

"Good afternoon, this is Dr. Ethan Surprenant. I wanted to check in after your little one's adjustment yesterday and let you know—"

"Doc!" she interrupted, her excitement spilling over. "It was wild! After you adjusted her, she had a huge blowout in her diaper. I was so worried—she hadn't been pooping, and I didn't know what to do!"

"Wow! Thank you for sharing—"

"And she's sleeping so deeply now, and feeding is so much easier. That was incredible! Thank you. It's like everything's just working now!"

"You're most welcome," I said, humbled by her gratitude. "It's amazing how well the body works when the nervous system is powered on effectively."

Her words, "It's like everything's just working now," stayed with me. That simple observation captures the remarkable power of a well-functioning nervous system. When communication between the brain and body is clear, even the most basic functions—sleeping, eating, digesting, and moving—can unfold naturally, just as they were designed to. This natural balance is made possible by the body's ability to maintain homeostasis.

Understanding Homeostasis

The body maintaining homeostasis is like a circus tightrope walker—constantly making subtle, precise adjustments to stay balanced high in the big top, even as the environment shifts around them. Similarly, the brain works behind the scenes to keep the body's internal environment stable, adapting quickly to external changes to maintain internal balance.

For example, when an infant's body temperature drops, their brain triggers muscle contractions, what we call shivering, to generate heat. When their body overheats, their brain activates sweat glands to cool the skin through evaporation. In the case of infection, the brain may raise body temperature to create a fever, helping to eliminate the threat, then follow with sweating to restore normal temperature.

Each of these adaptive responses is the body's way of walking the tightrope. This is homeostasis in action..

This process is vital for survival. It allows the nervous system to take in information from the infant's surroundings, integrate it into the brain's memory banks, and guide growth in a way that is best suited for the environment. While homeostasis has been functioning since conception, it becomes increasingly evident during infancy, as the baby interacts with the outside world for the first time.

Supporting the infant's ability to maintain homeostasis involves ensuring that the nervous system operates without interference and creating an environment that promotes healthy development.

A Baby's Four Jobs

As a parent—whether it's your first baby or not—it can be challenging to understand your infant's ability to maintain homeostasis when their primary form of communication is crying. Baby is hungry? Cry. Dirty diaper? Cry. Sleepy? Cry. A tag from the swaddle tickling their ear? Cry. Sometimes, a baby may even cry for no clear reason at all, simply trying to practice using their voice and build lung capacity. And while that might seem random, even this kind of crying serves a homeostatic purpose: strengthening the systems they'll rely on for breathing, vocalizing, and regulating stress.

So what is a parent to do when everything seems to come out as the same sound?

First, it's important to realize that babies always give feedback when something is off in their environment, both internal and external. Their cries are signals. They don't always point to something wrong, but they do always mean the baby is recognizing something has changed in their environment. Second, it helps to know what you're looking for. In infancy, a baby has four primary jobs: to eat, sleep, poop, and move. While these might sound like ordinary routines to us, they're actually some of the clearest reflections of how well the nervous system is functioning and how well the baby is maintaining internal balance. Each one of them comes with a unique cry from the infant. Understanding the jobs clearly, pairing them with your baby's unique cries allows for parents to actively differentiate between which of the four jobs needs attention when their baby does cry.

Each of the four jobs play a role in preserving homeostasis. If a baby can't nurse effectively, perhaps because they can't open their mouth wide enough or turn their head comfortably to one side, they won't receive the nutrients their growing brain and body depend on. If sleep is disrupted, they miss out on deep cellular repair and critical brain development that only happens during deep and REM sleep. If pooping becomes irregular, digestion slows down, toxins can build up, and inflammation may rise, further challenging the body's internal balance. And if the baby can't move freely or prefers to lie in just one position, their muscles, ligaments, and reflexes don't have the chance to develop in a coordinated, symmetrical way, which can create future challenges for motor development and posture.

When something interferes with one of these jobs, it's often the first clue that the nervous system is working harder than it ought to. We are going to take some time to understand the importance of these four jobs in maintaining homeostasis to help parents shift from feeling helpless to becoming active observers of their baby's well-being—and it lays the groundwork for how to support healthy neurodevelopment in the months and years ahead.

Sleep and Restoration: Growth Through Rest

Sleep is arguably the most important contributor to neurological development and to maintaining homeostasis. During sleep, a baby's body repairs itself, integrates new skills, and regulates its internal environment. Newborns require 16–18 hours of sleep per day, cycling through two primary sleep stages: REM sleep (Rapid Eye Movement) and NREM sleep (Non-Rapid Eye Movement). REM sleep is a lighter, active sleep stage where motor skills and memory are processed, while NREM sleep is the deeper stage responsible for clearing neurological waste and promoting cellular repair. Unlike adults, who spend about 20% of their sleep cycle in REM and take up to 90 minutes to enter it, infants begin their sleep in REM and spend nearly 50% of their total sleep time in this phase, meaning a baby's sleep cycle is half motor and memory training and half nervous system cleaning and repair.

If there are disruptions in the nervous system (like being stuck in a sympathetic neurologic tone), babies may struggle to stay asleep long enough to cycle through growth and repair. Without sufficient sleep, their ability to regulate internal processes, process new experiences, and recover from daily activity is compromised. Sleep disturbances can indicate underlying nervous system dysfunction, making it essential to support neurological balance to ensure deep, restorative sleep. When infants are able to sleep soundly, their brain and body can fully recover and continue developing as intended.

Feeding, Digestion, Excretion: Raw Materials for Growth

A well-fed baby has the energy and building blocks needed for growth and development. However, feeding is not just about consuming food—it also involves digesting, absorbing, and assimilating nutrients while efficiently excreting waste. This intricate balance is governed by a complex interplay of cranial and sacral nerves:

- **Cranial Nerves VII, IX, X, XI, XII:** Coordinate latching, sucking, and swallowing.
- **Cranial Nerve VIII:** Helps the baby orient spatially to locate the nipple.
- **Cranial Nerve X (Vagus):** Regulates digestion and nutrient absorption.
- **Sacral Plexus:** Controls the lower digestive tract and elimination process.

When the nervous system is balanced, these digestive processes work seamlessly. However, in about one-third of cases, mothers still report that their babies struggle with latch issues. Even when feeding appears successful, structural misalignments in the skull, upper cervical spine, or sacrum can disrupt digestion, leading to colic, constipation, or malabsorption. These challenges can deprive the baby of the building blocks needed for optimal growth.

Alternatively, in a neurologically sound infant, nutrients are broken down, absorbed, and distributed effectively, maintaining homeostasis. Unneeded nutrients are excreted, completing the cycle of efficient nutrient use and waste elimination and providing the infant with all the necessary nutritional building blocks for a life of health.

Movement: The Need for a Stable Framework

An infant's skeletal system is largely cartilage at birth, making it highly malleable and responsive to external forces. This flexibility allows for growth and adaptation, but it also makes proper alignment and movement essential for healthy development.

A key early milestone is tummy time, which introduces the infant to weight-bearing outside the womb. This activity strengthens muscles, promotes proper spinal curvature, and builds spatial awareness. It also ensures equal forces on the skull, preventing flat spots and supporting healthy cranial development.

Bones act as both levers for movement and protective structures. The cranial bones protect the brain, while the spinal column shields the spinal cord. These bones are soft and unfused at birth, allowing for optimal movement of the body and circulation of a solution created within the brain called cerebrospinal fluid (CSF). CSF delivers nutrients to the brain, removes waste, and supports neurological health. Proper CSF circulation depends on a smooth flow path through skull, spine, and nervous system. Do you remember where we mentioned that 99% of newborns show some dysfunction of the cranial bones, upper cervical spine, and sacrum? These are the main pumps for the CSF. While we won't get into the complete depths of how this CSF pump works here, the important point is this: misalignments in the skull and spine can disrupt the normal flow of this fluid and lead to accumulation of neurologic waste in the brain and hindering the speed of homeostatic responses.

Implications for Neurodevelopment

Because a baby's world revolves around sleeping, eating, pooping, and moving, these functions are profound indicators of the body's ability to maintain balance and regulate itself. When these foundational processes function smoothly, they reflect a nervous system that is clear, coordinated, and capable of guiding the body's growth and adaptation.

However, when disruptions occur in any of these areas, it is critical to consider neurological factors as potential root causes. Sleep disturbances may signal difficulty shifting into parasympathetic control. Feeding challenges may point to nerve interference in the head and upper neck. Colic or constipation can indicate Vagus nerve or sacral plexus dysfunction. Delays in motor milestones often suggest improper joint alignment affecting muscle activation.

By addressing these neurological factors early through tools like upper cervical chiropractic care and spinal alignment, parents can support their baby's ability to thrive and maintain homeostasis.

Transition to Toddlerhood

As infants master the essential tasks of sleeping, eating, pooping, and moving, they begin their transition into toddlerhood—a time defined by rapid neuroplasticity, exploration, and trial-and-error learning. This stage builds on the strong foundation laid during infancy, with every step, word, and new experience shaping critical brain connections. In the next chapter, we'll uncover how this dynamic period of growth and discovery sets the stage for speech, coordination, and problem-solving, and how parents can guide their child through the unique challenges and opportunities of toddlerhood.

Chapter 12

Toddlerhood

Understanding Neuroplasticity

Dr. Ethan

"Look at this!" my wife yelled from across the living room. I (Dr. Ethan) hurried over, startled—my wife is not one to yell unless it's important.

"What's going on?" I asked as she held her phone up to face me.

"Look! This is from the mom of the 2-year-old you adjusted a couple of days ago," she exclaimed.

I read the text on her screen: *Tell Ethan that this past week she started saying so many words! She's added so much to her vocabulary!*

The little girl had been struggling with vocal milestones and speech delays. Although she had been working with a speech therapist for months, progress had been minimal. She knew basic sign language and could understand what her parents were saying, but she couldn't communicate her own thoughts. There was a blockage preventing her brain from smoothly transitioning thoughts into spoken words. But now, that blockage was gone, and she had found her voice—a voice full of potential and hope for the future.

Repetitive Learning

Parents of children who have struggled to meet milestones can likely sympathize with the parents of that little girl. Few things are as stressful as seeing your child struggle without understanding the root of the problem—the *why* behind their challenges.

As babies transition into toddlerhood, their physical structure adapts in preparation for the upcoming season of exploratory falls, bumps, and bruises. Cranial sutures begin to harden and fuse, taking the once soft skull of a baby – protected only by mom and dad – into a hard object capable of protecting the brain from the consequences of adventure gone wrong. Spinal bone structures further ossify (transforming from cartilage to bone), offering better support and anchor points for developing muscles and ligaments, all while safeguarding nerves designed to extend the reach of the brain's instructions for development. Weight-bearing bones (legs, feet, arms, etc.) thicken as toddlers squat, jump, and run their way through these early years.

Along with the physical changes that occur in toddlerhood, this is a period of immense neurological growth. In fact, there is the largest jump in synaptogenesis (the amount of neurologic connections created) in the first 3 years of life. As toddlers' brains grow, they become naturally more investigative. *What happens when I push this cup off the table? What happens when I hit this metal pan? What happens when I slap this puddle on the table? What happens when I squeeze this egg really tight?* They become little scientists!

This investigative need is filled by many tiny moments of trial and error—children attempting small tasks, taking risks, failing, trying again, and repeating the process over and over. This is when the "why?" the "no" and the "I do it" show up. While this behavior can often frustrate parents, it serves an essential purpose, it drives the most important element of early brain development: neuroplasticity.

Neuroplasticity is the brain's remarkable ability to adapt and strengthen neural pathways through repetition. Whether it's throwing balls, climbing furniture, jumping, or practicing new words and sounds, these repeated actions refine the brain's control over movement, speech, and perception of the world. When the brain goes through neuroplastic changes, it makes the synaptic connections between nerves stronger, causes the nerves themselves to thicken, and, in these young toddler years, even recruits more of the nervous system to strengthen and refine each action.

It's not just that the nerve works more smoothly—it is physically building a stronger, thicker, and more robust neural pathway. Much like a muscle that becomes stronger and thicker with exercise, the physical nerves themselves are reinforced through repetition. Each clumsy attempt and every repeated effort contribute to building and solidifying these pathways. Over time, these changes transform tentative motions and hesitant speech into coordinated movement, clear communication, and growing mastery over their environment. And the changes made during toddlerhood become the foundation of lifelong skills and abilities—physically constructing the neurological framework for success later in life.

For toddlers with a smooth infancy (with consistent eating, sleeping, pooping, and growing), this phase often progresses with only minor setbacks—occasional illnesses, falls, and the inevitable bumps along the way. However, toddlers who experienced a difficult birth, early feeding challenges, consistent sleep disturbances, prolonged neurological stress, or unresolved structural dysfunctions during infancy may face compounded struggles. Unaddressed structural misalignments, particularly in the spine or cranial bones, can disrupt neuroplastic changes. These disruptions often manifest in critical areas like speech development, motor milestones, or sensory functions.

Speech Development and Neurological Coordination

Speech is one of the most significant milestones of toddlerhood, and one of the best reflections of the quality of neuroplasticity. It requires a finely tuned coordination between sensory input and motor output, all needing to be practiced over and over. Renowned public speaking expert., Vinh Giang, describes a person's voice as "their instrument." How many people have you met who are experts in music the first time they touch an instrument? Or even for the first year of practicing? I haven't met anyone like that. Toddlers are the same when learning to use their "instrument."

Speaking may seem simple because we do it all day without thinking, but it's actually an incredibly complex process. Every time your child hears a sound, tiny structures in the ear turn that sound into signals that travel through nerves into the brainstem, right near the upper neck, and then up into the parts of the brain that process language. From there, the brain decides how to respond and sends signals back down through nerves that control the lips, tongue, and jaw. At the same time, the child is watching the way other people's mouths move and matching those patterns to the sounds they hear.

This complex interplay between hearing, sight, and mouth movement is practiced thousands of times to allow the young child to observe sounds and translate them from visual cues into personal speech. The foundations for this began with infancy in observation of mom and dad speaking to the infant but this is the first time the infant's vocal muscles are strong enough to produce the observed and practiced sounds.

Tension or misalignment affecting the brainstem or cranial nerves can interfere with this intricate process, particularly speech production. This was precisely the case with the little girl at the beginning of the chapter. Her ability to understand speech was intact – she was attentive, practiced her mouth and tongue movements, listened well – but her brain and body could not coordinate effectively to produce spoken words. It was a communication problem along these nerve pathways. Once the interference in her nervous system was alleviated, communication between her brain and body improved, allowing her to speak and repeat sounds. These repetitions activated neuroplastic changes, which in turn fueled her rapid progress in speech development.

The same principle applies to other developmental milestones, such as walking and social skills. Structural misalignments or neurological disruptions can create barriers to progress in these areas. When these systems do not work harmoniously, children struggle to develop the essential skills needed for growth and adaptation.

Keys to Supporting Healthy Toddlerhood

Because toddlerhood is defined by rapid neuroplasticity, when a child faces structural or neurological challenges, the efficiency of creating neuroplastic changes can be disrupted. Addressing issues in neurologic function early is crucial in breaking the cycle of developmental delays and ensuring toddlers can reach their full potential.

Poor structural alignment can be a hindrance to the neuroplastic process. Tension on the brainstem and cranial nerves limits the potential for learning and practicing. Proper alignment of the cranial bones and upper cervical spine allows for intact and clear communication between the brain and body, creating the necessary conditions for speech, movement, and cognitive development. Equally important to structural alignment is the parental responsibility of providing toddlers with ample opportunities for play, exploration, and engagement. Parents should strike a balance between child-directed free-play and parent-directed activities. Through active learning with proper spinal alignment, children develop essential cognitive, social, and physical skills, reinforcing their ability to explore, adapt, and thrive.

Repetition and trial-and-error learning remain at the heart of toddlerhood, strengthening neural connections and preparing children for more advanced developmental milestones. However, as they transition into early childhood, new challenges emerge. The brain's adaptability is put to the test as external stressors, ranging from environmental toxins to emotional and immune challenges, begin to shape or hinder neurodevelopment in significant ways.

Transition to Early Childhood: Preparing for New Challenges

Next, we'll explore how chronic stress affects a child's immune system, emotional regulation, and cognitive growth during early childhood. Understanding how to navigate and minimize these stressors is essential to fostering resilience and unlocking the full potential of this critical stage of development. Let's move forward and examine how parents can support their child through the complexities of early childhood.

Chapter 13

Early Childhood

Fatigue and Frustration

Dr. Ethan

"He's regressed somehow," the young boy's father said, his voice heavy with concern. "His mom and I wish we had done things differently during his early years."

The boy was full of life, yet his stimming behaviors and inability to communicate verbally revealed the disarray in his nervous system.

"He *was* able to speak," the father continued, "and he was making good progress through his milestones. But then he got sick, went on antibiotics, got caught up on his shots, and... he just stopped progressing."

My heart sank. "I'm sure you did the best you could with the information you had at the time. Figuring out complex health problems isn't easy for first-time parents."

"Do you think there's anything you can do?"

"We'll do everything we can to find the root of the problem and work to correct it. The rest will depend on his nervous system."

The Effect of Early Chronic Stress

Early childhood is typically a time of wonder, exploration, and the rapid acquisition of skills as a result of children encountering more outside-the-home experiences. It's a time where a delicate and developing nervous system gets to experience the beginnings of adaptation and resilience. For healthy children, it's a phase marked by increasing independence, curiosity, and growth.

However, some children do not start in this healthy state. Leading up to this age, they may miss milestones, struggle with colic or constipation, and show behavioral issues often written off as the "terrible twos." As a result, early childhood—the preschool years from ages three to five—falls short of optimal development.

Still others, like the young boy in our story, start out seemingly fine, hitting milestones and showing emotional regulation. Then, a stressful event exposes cracks in the child's neurologic foundation, leading to sudden regression. Early childhood should be a time of growth—physically, socially, and cognitively. But for some children, it becomes a season of fatigue, frustration, and regression. Whether the struggle is failing to progress or suddenly regressing, one factor is always present: chronic stress.

Chronic stress, in this context, is best understood as the result of the unresolved accumulation of stressors over time. If you've ever watched a toddler build a block tower, you know how it goes. The blocks aren't stacked with perfect balance. They wobble, shift, and lean until eventually one more block causes the whole thing to topple. Chronic stress operates in a similar way. Sometimes it's obvious where the stress is coming from, such as excessive screen time, falls down stairs or off the couch, or food allergies. Other times the source is harder to see, like overscheduling without enough rest, repeated tumbles while learning to walk, or ongoing family conflict. In both sources, the effects of chronic stress ripple through every aspect of a child's life.

While adults under chronic stress may experience symptoms like fatigue, brain fog, and headaches, children exhibit symptoms of stress differently. Prolonged stress in a child can cause emotional dysregulation, chronic exhaustion, frequent infections, and hypersensitivity to stimuli such as sounds, lights, or crowded environments. This chronic stress can also manifest in cognitive delays, attention difficulties, social challenges, and motor delays. Over time, these symptoms are often grouped under common diagnoses like Attention-Deficit/Hyperactivity Disorder (ADHD), Autism Spectrum Disorder (ASD), or Sensory Processing Disorder (SPD). But these labels rarely address the underlying causes. Instead, these stressors pile up, placing a heavier burden on the nervous system. As the child grows and takes on more demands from their environment, the delays only increase. Unfortunately, many medical evaluations stop at these diagnoses and prescribe long-term medication without exploring the deeper "why" behind the symptoms.

Since, for many parents, early childhood is the first time they notice a significant departure from typical development—especially when observing their child among their peers at church, the park, playdates, or early group settings—it is crucial to recognize the drivers of chronic stress. Addressing these roots can improve or even resolve delays already present and decrease the chance of future developmental delays.

As we move forward, we'll explore the main factors that drive the accumulation of chronic stress in children, what can be done to stop the accumulation of stress, and the potential outlook of a healthy brain during this stage of development.

Emotional Overload

Imagine being a young child, just 3 to 5 years old, who has struggled with basic functions—sleeping, digesting food, and connecting socially—since birth. No matter what your parents do, you can't stay asleep, and when you do, nightmares or restless energy keep you from feeling rested. You wake up tired, and your parents still rush you through a morning routine you haven't quite grasped yet. Some of the meals that you eat make your stomach hurt, but you don't know why. You still haven't gone to the bathroom, your belly feels full of pressure, and you're gassy all the time. You're uncomfortable, yet your parents want you to greet people and play with other kids even though you haven't slept and your stomach aches. You feel bad but don't know how to explain it—and wouldn't know where to begin anyway. After all, you don't have many words yet. The stress builds, compounding the struggles you already carried as an infant, pushing your body further into dysfunction.

This situation is all too common for children today. Each daily activity—getting dressed, eating breakfast, going out to play—seems normal on its own. After all, these are things every child does. But when the pace is rushed, the instructions seem harsh, and empathy is missing in the process, the weight on a child's nervous system becomes extraordinary. Instead of building resilience, these everyday moments lock the body into a persistent state of stress.

When stress becomes chronic, the nervous system can get trapped in sympathetic dominance—fight-or-flight stuck in overdrive. This is especially concerning for children whose systems are still developing and may already be vulnerable from a difficult infancy or toddlerhood. As we discussed in the Emotional Fortitude chapter, living in this state means the body behaves as though it's under constant attack. Learning and focus are suppressed, the immune system is weakened, energy reserves run dry, and digestion falters, which leads to malnourishment and poor growth.

A child stuck here is essentially running from an internal bear that never goes away. Without relief, the body cannot shift into the parasympathetic state required for rest, healing, and growth. As Dr. Bruce Lipton, Ph.D., explains in The Biology of Belief: "You can't be in growth and protection at the same time." If the everyday demands of life consistently overwhelm a child's nervous system, the result is not growth, but survival.

Structural Stress

Earlier in this book, we discussed how structural misalignments in the cranial bones, upper cervical spine, or sacrum can interfere with digestion, delay milestones, and weaken vagus nerve function. In early childhood, these same misalignments begin to create even more visible effects.

A structural misalignment alters the way the body reports information back to the brain. Joint position, ligament tension, muscle tone, and organ function all send constant updates through the nervous system. When alignment is off, those signals become distorted. This disruption is called disafferentation. It means the brain is no longer receiving an accurate picture of what is happening inside the body.

When the brain is fed faulty input, it often interprets it as a sign of danger. The body shifts into stress mode, even when no real threat exists. Muscles stay tight, blood flow prioritizes survival, and the nervous system gets stuck in fight-or-flight. Over time, this drains energy that should be going toward growth, learning, and repair.

Parents may notice this stress pattern in ways that don't immediately appear structural. A child may be clumsy, bump into objects, or struggle with coordination. They may have ongoing stomachaches, restless sleep, or hypersensitivity to sound or touch. In some cases, the brain's attempt to self-regulate these faulty signals shows up as repetitive, stimming-type behaviors like those commonly associated with neurodevelopmental disorders like ASD. The stimming happens because the nervous system is searching for order in the middle of scrambled input, and the child's outward behaviors reflect that effort.

The important point is this: even without obvious external stressors, misalignments can create a constant stream of false alarms within the nervous system. For the child, it feels as if their body is never fully at rest. This internal stress loop compounds the burden of chronic stress and keeps them from accessing the calm, parasympathetic state required for healthy neurodevelopment.

Immune Challenges

Early childhood is when children begin to stretch beyond the safety of home and engage more actively with their environment. Preschool, playdates, church nurseries, and park outings expose them to a constant stream of new people, new surroundings, and, inevitably, new germs.

For a child with a strong, well-functioning immune system, these exposures aren't just normal—they're healthy. Each cold, stomach bug, or mild fever becomes a training exercise, giving the body practice at mounting an appropriate defense and then standing down once the threat has passed. This is how resilience is built.

But for children already worn down by disrupted sleep, poor nutrition, or prolonged sympathetic dominance, this process doesn't unfold the way it should. Parents quickly learn that their child doesn't "just get over things." What should be a short-lived cold turns into a drawn-out ordeal. Infections like strep throat appear again and again, despite repeated treatments. When a fever does arise, it is often suppressed with over-the-counter medication before the body has a chance to use that fever as a powerful, natural weapon to "bake out" infection. Instead of helping, this stunts the immune system's effectiveness and leaves the child more vulnerable to the next illness.

Over time, this cycle escalates. Parents find themselves in an ENT's office after multiple infections, getting recommendations for surgical solutions like tonsillectomies or adenoidectomies. While these procedures can bring short-term relief, it's important to recognize that tonsils and adenoids are not useless structures. They are part of the body's immune surveillance system, designed to detect and fight pathogens entering through the mouth and nose. Their removal may reduce infections in the short run, but it also strips away part of the immune system's natural defense line—another example of trading long-term resilience for short-term symptom relief.

For many families, antibiotics remain the most common intervention. And while antibiotics can be lifesaving, frequent or broad-spectrum use often brings unintended consequences. Antibiotics don't discriminate: while they kill harmful bacteria, they also wipe out the beneficial bacteria in the gut that regulate digestion, immunity, and even mood and behavior. This is the "friendly fire" effect—an attempt to take down the enemy that ends up damaging your own defenses.

The gut is sometimes called the "second brain," and with good reason. The trillions of microbes in the gut don't just help break down food; they send constant feedback to the nervous system about the state of the body. When healthy bacteria are destroyed and not replenished, the signals that travel from the gut to the brain become distorted or incomplete. Just as a structural misalignment leads to disafferentation, a disrupted microbiome creates its own form of disafferentation. The brain receives "bad reports," and its ability to coordinate a proper immune or healing response is weakened.

This friendly fire effect wouldn't be as destructive if antibiotics were consistently paired with deliberate efforts to restore gut health. Probiotic supplements, or fermented foods like yogurt, kefir, sauerkraut, or kimchi, can help repopulate the microbiome and rebuild resilience. But in practice, this step is rarely recommended. The child is left with a compromised gut, weakened digestion, inefficient nutrient absorption, greater inflammation, and impaired gut-brain communication. Over time, the result is a vicious cycle: more illness, more antibiotics, greater gut disruption, and deeper developmental delays.

The consequences reach far beyond missed preschool days or frequent doctor visits. A child who is sick more often than well loses crucial opportunities for play, exploration, and social interaction—the very experiences that drive neurodevelopment in early childhood. Instead of moving forward, they are repeatedly pulled backward, trapped in a survival loop where the immune system never fully regains its strength.

Restoring Balance and Building Lasting Resilience

The chronic stress patterns we have explored—emotional overload, structural misalignments, and immune suppression—are not separate issues, but interconnected pieces of the same cycle. At the center is sympathetic dominance: a nervous system locked in survival mode, unable to access the calm, restorative parasympathetic state that fuels growth and healing. Left unchecked, this cycle weakens immunity, scrambles communication between the brain and body, and erodes emotional stability. Over time, the cumulative burden increases the likelihood of developmental delays and contributes to the expression of neurodevelopmental disorders such as ADHD, ASD, or SPD.

Breaking this cycle begins with decreasing sympathetic tone and restoring proper balance within the nervous system. When structural misalignments are corrected and neural tension is resolved, the brain can once again receive accurate feedback from the body. Joint position, ligament and muscle tension, organ function, and even gut microbiome activity all send clear, reliable signals. This accurate input allows the brain to coordinate responses with precision—turning off the stress alarm when no danger exists and activating parasympathetic processes when healing, digestion, or recovery are needed.

As parasympathetic function is restored, the changes are often striking. Sleep becomes deeper and more restorative. Digestion and nutrient absorption improve, fueling both body and brain. Immune responses strengthen, reducing the frequency and duration of infections. Emotional fortitude builds, with children displaying greater adaptability, fewer meltdowns, and an increased ability to engage socially. With the nervous system operating as it was designed, the body is no longer trapped in survival mode—it is free to grow, learn, and thrive.

The most powerful outcome of addressing these issues at their root is not simply the reduction of symptoms but the reinforcement of resilience. By lowering chronic stress, strengthening immunity, and ensuring clear brain–body communication, parents can help their children lay a neurological foundation that protects against the development of long-term disorders.

Children whose nervous systems regain balance often surprise their parents with just how much potential was waiting beneath the surface. Improvements in sleep, focus, emotional regulation, and immune strength are not random "miracles"—they are the natural result of a body freed from interference, finally able to function the way it was designed.

Navigating the Grade School Years

Early childhood is a season of rapid growth, but as we've seen, it can also be weighed down by chronic stress when emotional overload, structural misalignments, and immune challenges remain unresolved.

As I mentioned, these patterns don't simply fade with age—they compound. By the time a child reaches grade school, the nervous system is asked to handle even greater demands while still carrying the weight of early dysfunction.

The classroom introduces new pressures: sustained academic focus, navigating peer relationships, and longer separations from parents. These challenges do not create problems by themselves, but they magnify what is already happening inside a child's body and mind. Struggles with attention, emotional regulation, immune resilience, and social confidence often become more visible, leaving children overwhelmed and parents searching for answers.

In the next chapter, we'll explore how the grade school years push a child's nervous system to adapt to an entirely new environment. We'll uncover why symptoms like poor concentration, emotional outbursts, and recurrent illnesses often emerge more strongly during this time— and how they reflect deeper patterns of stress within the body. Most importantly, we'll look at how addressing the root causes can shift a child's trajectory, helping them thrive rather than simply cope as they face the academic and social challenges of these formative years.

Chapter 14

Grade School Years

Social and Academic Demands

Dr. Ethan

"We see why your son has been struggling in school," the doctor began, addressing the visibly tired mother of three. "Do you see these scans? The red means he has excessive tension in the upper neck on the right side, and the mid-back on the left side. And this dot here? This is his heart rate variability. It's showing that his autonomic nervous system is under intense stress and has been for some time."

I stood quietly, observing as I shadowed a Pediatric and Upper Cervical doctor during my last few months in chiropractic school. So many children, stuck in chronic stress overload, had come to the office during my time there. This young boy was no different—a 6th grader who had been helping care for his little siblings, including a non-verbal autistic sister. He had taken on responsibilities far beyond his years. The bags under his eyes told the story of sleepless nights. His slouched posture spoke of burdens too heavy for his young shoulders to carry.

"The good news is this," the doctor continued, "his ADHD, frequent illnesses, and the stress on his nervous system are all connected. If we address the root of the problem, he'll be able to bounce back."

"But I don't want you and Dad to have to spend all that money," the young boy said softly, glancing up at his mom with tired eyes. My heart sank. Even in his exhaustion, he was putting his family first.

"It's okay, baby," his mother replied, her voice a mix of sadness and deep appreciation. "Dad and I will take care of it. We want you to be healthy too."

Although I didn't get to observe the full course of care, I did see the early stages of the young man's treatment. Even within a few weeks, his transformation was remarkable. His eyes regained their sparkle, his posture improved, and he looked rested. Though the stresses in his life remained, he had clearly become more resilient to them. His nervous system was beginning to function as it should, allowing him to adapt and thrive.

The Past Sets Up the Future

The grade school years mark a transformative stage in a child's life, as they face increasing cognitive, social, and emotional demands. Children begin spending more time away from the direct oversight of their parents—at school, with friends, playing sports, and engaging in other activities.

For some children, this period fosters resilience, adaptability, and growth. For others, like the young boy in the story, it becomes a daily battle against fatigue, frustration, and seemingly insurmountable challenges, despite otherwise supportive environments.

As parents, the signs can feel confusing at first. A child who seems healthy may suddenly begin to struggle with things like staying focused, managing their emotions, or keeping up with sleep. Skills that once seemed mastered may slip backwards. Illnesses may become more frequent, or friendships may start to feel harder to navigate. These are the very challenges we'll explore next—not as isolated problems, but as connected expressions of how a child's nervous system is adapting under pressure.

Difficulty Focusing

For many families, focus issues are the first challenge that stands out in the grade school years. In toddlerhood, short attention spans are often excused as "just being a kid" or "they're too little to focus." By the teenage years, however, the same behaviors often draw frustration, resentment, or even offhand comments that sting—remarks spoken directly to the teen or about them within earshot. Those words can plant seeds of self-doubt and negative self-talk. In grade school, the gap between what a child can manage and what school requires becomes obvious: sitting still, following directions, and sustaining attention for 30–40 minutes at a time. If a child has never practiced self-discipline at home—like finishing a puzzle, playing quietly, or focusing on a single task without interruption—school quickly exposes the struggle.

At the same time, this is often the stage when children begin to experience large amounts of unregulated screen time—whether through TV, computer games at school, social media, or video games at home. Screens themselves aren't inherently bad; in fact, certain video games or educational programs can be beneficial. The challenge comes when use is unstructured and unrestricted. Research consistently shows a clear divide: children with less than two hours of screen exposure per day fare much better than those logging four, six, or even more hours. Today, even school environments and libraries are introducing more screen-based activities, meaning kids may spend hours in front of a screen before they ever get home. By the time they add after-school entertainment, their nervous system is flooded with stimulation it cannot fully process. The result is overwhelm—a brain trained to expect constant dopamine spikes, leaving children stuck in stress mode with little opportunity to shift into calm focus or true rest.

Emotional Outbursts or Withdrawal

Emotional struggles often surface in grade school because this is the first time children are regularly exposed to two very different worlds: home and school. At home, they may have one rhythm of meals, routines, and expectations. At school, they encounter a different schedule, different rules, and—most importantly—different ideas. For the first time, a child might hear something from a teacher or peer that contradicts what they've always been taught at home. That internal clash, known as cognitive dissonance, can be deeply unsettling for a developing brain. Toddlers simply repeat new information without much thought, but grade schoolers begin to wrestle with what's true and whom to trust. When two "trusted voices" collide, frustration often erupts as emotional outbursts, or, on the other end, withdrawal.

This tug-of-war only deepens when children feel the need to adopt different versions of themselves for home and school. Many will hold it together all day in the classroom—sitting still, following rules, and suppressing their natural energy—only to release it all when they walk through the front door. If the home doesn't feel like a safe space to unload those bottled-up emotions, the incongruence grows even greater. Over time, the mismatch between environments and expectations overwhelms a child's nervous system, leaving them oscillating between explosive reactions and complete shutdown. These behaviors aren't signs of defiance or poor character; they're the visible signals of a child struggling to reconcile competing worlds.

Sleep Disturbances

Back in the infancy chapter, we talked about the four primary jobs of a baby—eat, sleep, poop, and grow. Sleep is still just as essential for a grade school child because growth and brain development are still in full swing. Yet, this is also the age when sleep problems often begin to show. Children spend long hours in classrooms with limited movement, sometimes going days without physical education or outdoor play. Their natural energy has nowhere to go. Just as adults know the difference between falling into bed after an active day versus tossing and turning after a sedentary one, kids also struggle when their energy isn't released. The buildup makes it harder to fall asleep, stay asleep, and wake restored.

The problem compounds when earlier sleep difficulties—rooted in infancy—carry forward into these years. Add in late nights on screens, homework that stretches into the evening, and school schedules that demand early wake-up times, and the nervous system is pulled further out of rhythm. Parents may hesitate to set firm bedtime routines, not wanting to "limit" their child's freedom, but without that structure, sleep debt grows quickly. The result is more than just a tired child— learning suffers because the brain doesn't get the deep, restorative rest needed to cement the lessons of the day. Over time, poor sleep leaves children running on fumes, making every other challenge—focus, emotions, and even immunity—harder to manage.

Frequent Illnesses

Grade school is also the season when children seem to "catch everything." The reason isn't just bad luck—it's exposure. For the first time, kids are in close daily contact with dozens of peers, many of whom come to school with mild coughs or runny noses. A germ that barely slows one child down may take stronger hold in another who hasn't encountered it before. When you layer this higher exposure on top of a nervous system already taxed by poor sleep, excess screen stimulation, or emotional stress, the immune system simply has less capacity to fight back.

On top of that, most children in this age range have followed the standard vaccine schedule and may also face repeated antibiotic use for common infections. While this book isn't a debate on vaccines (see the appendices for more information), it's important to recognize the overall effect: the developing immune system is being asked to manage an increasing load of stressors—from vaccines, from pathogens, from medications, and from lifestyle. If recovery time is short or incomplete, one illness often stacks on top of another. Over time, the lack of recovery leaves children more vulnerable because their immune defenses never had had the chance to fully reset and build resilience.

Social Withdrawal and Regression in Skills

When focus, sleep, and physical health are already compromised, the social side of childhood rarely escapes untouched. A child who misses school often because of illness, or who can't keep up academically due to fatigue and poor concentration, naturally struggles to stay connected with peers. They may fall behind in shared experiences, even small things like learning new slang or keeping up with playground games. Because children are still developing empathy, peers can sometimes ridicule instead of support, and those repeated social blows wear heavily on a child's confidence. The result is often withdrawal—pulling back from friendships, group play, or even classroom participation—further reducing opportunities to build the regulation and resilience that come through healthy relationships.

In the most sensitive children—especially those already navigating ADHD, autism, or other developmental disorders—these pressures can become even more pronounced. And when the nervous system is under chronic stress, it sometimes reverts to earlier, simpler patterns as a coping mechanism. This regression may look like a return to bedwetting, constipation from withholding behaviors at school, or even change in previously established speech patterns. While this cycle can feel discouraging, it's important to recognize that it's not permanent. With consistent habits at home that support regulation—and, when needed, the right kind of clinical care—the nervous system can regain adaptability. When that happens, both social growth and developmental progress can be restored.

Building A Child's Resilience

If your child is experiencing these challenges—difficulty focusing, emotional outbursts, sleep disturbances, frequent illnesses, or social withdrawal—it's important to recognize that these are not isolated events or sudden shifts in how their body functions. These symptoms are evidence of a deeper, cumulative pattern of neurodevelopmental challenges that may have begun as early as birth or even during prenatal development. Parents often try to tackle these issues one by one—symptom by symptom or condition by condition—but without addressing the root causes, long-term change often remains elusive.

That's why we've walked through every stage of development leading to this point. Each chapter has emphasized how the compounding effects of early influences—both positive and negative—build the foundation for a child's health and neurodevelopment. We explored the critical role of the Six Pillars of Health during pregnancy and how challenges like C-sections, forceps delivery, or induced labor can introduce early strain. We examined how infancy often reveals the first signs of neurological dysfunction through symptoms like feeding difficulties, sleeping difficulties, delayed motor milestones, or colic. In toddlerhood, we showed how neurodevelopment relies on repetition and exploration. However, any neurological interference from earlier stages can hinder the speech and movement patterns necessary for building a strong foundation for later growth. And in early childhood we discussed how emotional and structural stress drive a fight-or-flight response, suppressing the immune system leading to a cycle of immunosuppression and potential neurodevelopmental disorders.

The great news is that there is hope for change even at these grade school ages, even if the problem has persisted since birth. Just like the story of the young boy with ADHD, chronic sickness, and stress, whose parents restored his nervous system's health through targeted care, your child's story can also shift. Once the deeper structural and neurological issues were addressed, that boy's life began to transform—and so can your child's.

So many of the neurodevelopmental challenges children face are rooted in foundational, neurologic issues that are often overlooked by both conventional medicine and holistic approaches. When the root causes like structural strain or chronic nervous system overload are addressed, the body's ability to heal and adapt is restored, and real, lasting change becomes possible.

When your child begins to struggle in school—meltdowns, emotional outbursts, or difficulty focusing—it's often not simply because school is "too hard" for them. Often, these challenges arise because there is already so much happening inside their body and nervous system. The additional demands of school and social interactions become the final straw that tips them over the edge. It's like the straw that breaks the camel's back—they simply cannot adapt any more.

This is why understanding your child's neurodevelopment and how to address these deeper issues is crucial. The pressures of grade school can magnify unresolved challenges, but with the right tools and insights, you can help your child build the resilience they need to thrive.

Becoming Teenagers

As children transition from grade school into adolescence, the stakes grow higher. The teenage years introduce new complexities: hormonal changes that magnify existing strengths or struggles, increased social pressures, and the desire for independence. These factors can amplify unresolved challenges from earlier stages, leading to intensified emotional turbulence, mental health concerns, and physical symptoms.

In the next chapter, we'll explore how the teenage years represent a pivotal period of neurodevelopment. You'll learn how hormones interact with the nervous system and why unresolved stressors often resurface in more dramatic ways during this stage. Let's uncover how you can support your teenager's growth and resilience as they navigate the unique challenges of adolescence.

Chapter 15

Teenage Years

Exhaustion and Emotional Erosion

Dr. Ethan

"I haven't had this much energy since before high school!" For 13 long years, this creative, energetic, and uplifting man had felt his potential stolen from him.

"That's amazing! And how did your first day back at work go?" I asked.

"Incredible! I actually felt good. I even had energy afterward. I'm thinking about getting back to drawing, exercising—maybe even dancing again. The negative thoughts are quieter now."

As a teenager, he had a passion for art, acting, martial arts, and an unstoppable drive for life. But the stressors of early childhood and adolescence had worn him down over time. Depression and anxiety crept in, dimming his creativity and motivation. Negativity became a constant shadow, robbing him of joy and progress.

But he sought answers. He refused to accept his state of exhaustion and frustration as permanent. By addressing the root causes of his struggles, he began to regain control over his nervous system and, with it, his life. Slowly but surely, his mind became clearer, his body stronger, and his spirit more resilient. He was reclaiming his sense of self, laying the foundation for a healthier, brighter future.

Being A Teen Is Neurologically Tough

The teenage years are notorious for their emotional ups and downs, filled with new experiences, identity exploration, and a growing desire for independence. For parents, this period can feel like navigating a rollercoaster. But when the challenges of adolescence go beyond normal turbulence—when teens are perpetually exhausted, frequently irritable, and disengaged from activities they once loved—it's often a sign of deeper neurological and physiological struggles.

These struggles are rarely just "teenage rebellion." Instead, they are the compounded effects of years of unresolved stress manifesting as profound exhaustion and emotional erosion. For some teens, this can mean living in a constant state of "survival mode," where joy and motivation feel out of reach.

The HPA Axis and the Stress Response

As the body transitions from childhood to adulthood, the hormonal changes of puberty amplify existing physiological patterns. Puberty acts as a magnifier, intensifying what's already present, whether it's healthy physiology or underlying stress and dysregulation.

At the heart of the body's ability to manage stress lies the hypothalamic-pituitary-adrenal (HPA) axis, an intricate system designed to adapt to and recover from stress. The HPA axis functions like a relay team, with three key players working together to regulate the body's stress response:

The Hypothalamus: The Monitoring System

The hypothalamus constantly monitors the body's internal and external environment for signs of stress or imbalance, such as danger, illness, or emotional strain. It acts as the body's alarm system, activating when a threat is detected. Upon recognizing a stressor, the hypothalamus sends a signal to the pituitary gland to initiate the stress response.

The Pituitary Gland: The Dispatcher

The pituitary gland receives the signal from the hypothalamus and acts as the body's dispatcher, sending out adrenocorticotropic hormone (ACTH) through the bloodstream. ACTH signals the adrenal glands to release stress hormones. While the pituitary also oversees other hormones like growth hormone and oxytocin, chronic stress diverts the pituitary's focus, throwing the entire hormonal system out of balance.

The Adrenal Glands: The Action Team

The adrenal glands, located above the kidneys, respond to ACTH by releasing stress hormones such as cortisol and adrenaline. These hormones prepare the body to react to stress: increasing heart rate, sharpening reflexes, and mobilizing energy. Once the stressor is resolved, the adrenal glands signal the hypothalamus to deactivate the alarm, allowing the system to return to balance.

Together, the HPA axis functions like emergency services in the event of a fire. The hypothalamus detects the fire and calls for help. The pituitary gland coordinates the response. The adrenal glands act quickly to put out the flames.

Under normal circumstances, this process resolves stress and restores balance. However, when stress becomes chronic—due to unresolved trauma, structural misalignments, or lifestyle factors—the HPA axis remains in overdrive. The result is a body stuck in fight-or-flight mode, unable to rest, recover, or properly adapt to its environment.

Hormonal Dysregulation in Teens

The teenage years introduce an added layer of complexity to the body's stress response system. Up until this point, the hormones released in the body were mostly focused on connection, growth, and neuroplastic change. But now, puberty and the hormonal shifts essential for physical development, growth, independence, and reproduction depend on a well-functioning HPA axis. When the body is locked in a state of chronic stress, it struggles to process and adapt to life's demands. This overload overwhelms the system and diverts resources away from critical growth and developmental processes.

Take, for example, the relationship between cortisol and estrogen. Most people think of cortisol only as the "stress hormone," but it also helps regulate blood sugar, inflammation, blood pressure, and sleep patterns. Estrogen, commonly associated with menstruation and female puberty, is integral in bone and muscle health, blood flow and circulation, cholesterol regulation, collagen production, and focus. Both hormones, estrogen and cortisol, share the same precursor molecule (a molecule which is made on the way to the final product), but under conditions of high stress, the body prioritizes cortisol production over estrogen. This imbalance leaves the body deficient in the estrogen needed for proper development. This can potentially delay puberty, disrupt mood regulation, and impair reproductive health. Similarly, in boys, chronic stress can suppress testosterone production, affecting physical strength, energy levels, and emotional stability.

The amplified demands of adolescence, such as academic pressures, social challenges, and the drive for independence, place additional strain on the HPA axis. Under normal circumstances, this system allows the body to recover from stress and maintain balance. However, when stress becomes chronic—whether from unresolved trauma, structural misalignments, or environmental influences—the HPA axis becomes overwhelmed. This keeps the body in a prolonged fight-or-flight state, unable to return to equilibrium.

For teenagers, this dysregulation often manifests as:
- Increased irritability and mood swings
- Emotional withdrawal or apathy
- Difficulty experiencing joy or connection
- Physical and cognitive exhaustion

These symptoms create a self-reinforcing downward spiral. Teens may withdraw from school, friendships, and hobbies, becoming disengaged and further isolated. For parents, this can be an especially painful experience as they watch their child struggle to meet the growing demands of adolescence while feeling powerless to help.

The Craniocervical Junction and Stress Regulation

The craniocervical junction (CCJ), which Dr. Chris mentioned in earlier chapters, plays a critical role in regulating the body's stress response and ensuring the proper functioning of the HPA axis. It serves as a gateway for hormonal signaling and transmission, facilitating the communication between the brain and the body. As such, it is a key intersection for hormone function and distribution.

The vertebral and carotid arteries, which supply oxygen and vital nutrients to the brain, including the hypothalamus, pass through the CCJ. Positioned in front of the CCJ is the jugular vein, the primary vein responsible for draining blood from the brain. Together, these structures control the movement of blood to and from the brain, carrying the hormones produced in the pituitary gland to the rest of the body.

Additionally, the Vagus nerve passes through the craniocervical junction, extending downward to innervate vital organs (heart, lungs, kidneys, liver) and regulate hormonal activity in the adrenal glands. A properly functioning Vagus nerve ensures balanced hormonal regulation and a healthy stress response.

For these blood vessels and nerves to perform their functions effectively, they require a clear pathway through the craniocervical junction. However, when the CCJ is misaligned, a commonly overlooked issue in the teenage population, it can create interference in these pathways, disrupting the body's ability to adapt to and recover from stress. This misalignment limits the communication between the brain and body, leading to a cascade of challenges, including diminished hormone regulation and a weakened ability to return to a state of equilibrium after stress.

In addition to the symptoms of hormone dysregulation mentioned earlier, this dysfunction can lead to headaches, migraines, and brain fog. These are hallmarks of a nervous system that is struggling to keep up with the heightened demands of adolescence. Addressing CCJ misalignments can restore critical pathways for blood flow and nerve signaling, allowing the body to function as intended and reducing the overwhelming symptoms of stress that many adolescents face.

Compounding Effects Grow

The teenage years are a pivotal stage when the neurologic patterns reinforced since infancy and childhood begin to solidify, making any underlying dysfunction more difficult to undo. As teenagers encounter less predictable influences (high school, the workplace, social gatherings), the chances of negative health patterns becoming more complex and multifaceted increase. Issues that began earlier in life, whether in the structural, nutritional, emotional, mental, chemical, or neurologic pillars of health, often compound during this time. The more pillars that have been neglected, the more deeply these maladaptive patterns become embedded, and the greater the challenge of restoring balance and healing.

Even if some of these underlying dysfunctions have been going on throughout their childhood, it is still possible as a teenager to change the trajectory, unwind the damage, and set the teenager on a path toward strength, resilience, and lasting health into adulthood.

Chapter 16

Adulthood

Lingering Effects of Dysregulation

Dr. Ethan

"I was about seven years old when it started. I got really sick back then and thought it would pass. But I never really got fully better. I always had brain fog, ear infections, and just felt out of sorts. It wasn't until a few years ago, after an accident, that I was finally diagnosed with Chronic Lyme Disease. I've tried so many things, but I need help that lasts."

This man's story was heavy, a lifetime of compounding neurological challenges stacking higher and higher since childhood. His health struggles impacted his relationships, derailed his career, and left him unable to maintain a consistent fitness routine. No matter what he tried, lasting resolution remained elusive. He deeply desired more from life, but his body couldn't keep up.

Fast forward three months. The same man, once exhausted from years of chronic stress and neurological dysregulation, walked into the office with a renewed sense of purpose. "I feel like I finally have my life back," he said. After 3 months of care, his ability to adapt to life's stressors had improved, his energy had returned, and his hope for the future had been restored. It was a big step forward from where he started.

Cumulative Dysregulation

The long-lasting effects of childhood dysregulation are far more common than most people realize. According to the CDC, one in six adults has experienced some form of childhood trauma that contributed to chronic illness in adulthood. Even more striking, five of the ten leading causes of death in adults are linked to adverse childhood experiences. The factors that shape our health are cumulative —events, habits, decisions, and exposures stack over time to either support or undermine our well-being.

Adulthood is the culmination of a lifetime of influences beginning back as far as preconception. This could be something that affects one of your adult children, or it could be something that even affects you. The health of your parents, their diet, toxin exposures, and stress management all contributed to your early neurodevelopment. From the prenatal environment to the birth process and the formative years of childhood, these experiences established the foundation for lifelong health.

During prenatal development, the nervous system formed in direct response to the mother's nutrition, stress chemistry, toxic load, and structural health. A supportive womb environment would have fostered resilience, while poor inputs during this stage could have left vulnerabilities before birth. The birth process itself was designed to "switch on" neurologic, hormonal, and structural systems. But if that process was disrupted or overly forceful, the strain may have carried forward into life outside the womb.

Infancy was the first real test. In those months, the body's ability to sleep, eat, digest, and move revealed how clearly the brain and body were communicating—or whether interference was already present. For many adults, the struggles they see in their children, or perhaps recall from their own earliest years, began showing here in subtle but telling ways.

When someone was a toddler, their brain underwent one of the greatest bursts of neuroplastic change in life. Every repetition of words, steps, and play physically shaped the nervous system, building stronger pathways and deeper reserves of adaptability. Yet if unresolved stress or structural strain carried over from earlier years, those gains may have been muted—slowing speech, motor coordination, or sensory development.

In early childhood, chronic stress became the great disruptor. If a child was burdened by repeated illnesses, disrupted sleep, or constant tension at home, their nervous system may have been pulled into survival mode. Instead of thriving in a season meant for physical, social, and cognitive growth, they may have been learning how to simply get by—trading resilience for fatigue, focus for frustration. Some of you may have seen this unfold in your own families.

By the grade school years, the added pressures of academics, social dynamics, and new responsibilities began to magnify what was already happening inside. If the nervous system had been carrying too much stress, challenges with concentration, emotional regulation, or frequent illness may have become more noticeable, setting patterns that carried forward.

Adolescence then amplified everything further. Puberty acted like a magnifying glass, intensifying both strengths and struggles. For many, this meant that unresolved stress from earlier years resurfaced more dramatically, showing up as exhaustion, mood swings, or hormonal dysregulation. Structural strain at the craniocervical junction, combined with a stressed system already under pressure, may have left the body feeling stuck in survival mode—unable to fully recover, adapt, or reset.

By the time someone reaches adulthood, the symptoms they or their children struggle with today often have their roots in these earlier developmental challenges. What began as subtle stressors or missed milestones in the early years may now appear as persistent patterns of dysfunction.

The signs of nervous system dysregulation in adults can show up in many ways, including:

- Chronic stress, anxiety, or depression
- Digestive issues and poor nutrient absorption

- Back and neck pain
- Migraines and headaches
- Brain fog and cognitive decline
- Chronic fatigue and low energy
- Dysautonomia (including POTS)
- Occipital or trigeminal neuralgia

Because these symptoms are so common, society has started to see them as "normal." But there is nothing normal about chronic pain, constant fatigue, or recurring headaches. The only thing that is truly normal is health itself. These symptoms are signs that something deeper is out of balance in the body. And when dysregulation becomes severe, the body may lose its ability to heal on its own. At that point, many people find themselves relying heavily on medications to manage symptoms—sometimes to the extent of overuse or dependency. What's most important, though, is not simply recognizing the condition itself, but uncovering the true root of the problem—both where it shows up today and where it first began, often reaching back to childhood experiences that set the stage for lifelong patterns of health or dysfunction.

The Slowdown of Neurodevelopment in Adulthood

Structural issues, particularly in the adult spine, are a commonly overlooked factor in ongoing dysregulation. Misalignments in the Craniocervical junction (CCJ) can:

- Limit blood flow into the brain, reducing oxygen and nutrient delivery.
- Slow blood flow out of the brain, increasing intracranial pressure.
- Disrupt cerebrospinal fluid (CSF) flow, impairing waste removal.
- Directly interfere with brainstem function, leaving the autonomic nervous system stuck in fight-or-flight mode.
- Interfere with nerve pathways from the body to the brain, causing systemic dysfunctions in primary body systems such as digestion, cardiovascular function, and immune response.

These disruptions contribute to chronic health issues such as poor digestion, emotional dysregulation, chronic pain, and an inability to recover from stress. In the most severe circumstances, they can even lead to early neurodegeneration. This means that unresolved structural issues and other factors can actually cause the brain to break down earlier than it otherwise would. Not only does this inhibit neurodevelopment, but once the aggressive growth stages of life have passed, unresolved issues can accelerate the brain's decline.

While the brain retains neuroplasticity in adulthood, the speed in which the brain changes slows down. Most major neural pathways have already been established by this stage, meaning the habits and structures formed in childhood have a profound impact on an adult's ability to thrive. This slower rate of adaptation makes reversing long-standing dysregulation more challenging, but not impossible.

Reversing Course in Adulthood

Despite the challenges of reversing long-standing dysregulation, adulthood still presents an opportunity for neurological change. Addressing key pillars of health can significantly improve your quality of life. Here's some practical steps:

- **Nutritional Saturation**: Prioritize nutrient-dense foods to support energy production and cellular repair. Addressing deficiencies can restore vitality and improve function.
- **Chemical Purity**: Reduce toxin exposures and detoxify the body to enhance brain clarity, gut health, and overall vitality. As you clean up the body, every system works more efficiently and adapts faster.
- **Structural Stability**: Seek proper spinal alignment through care from Upper Cervical Chiropractors or other specialists. Movement and exercise with an interference-free nervous system also promotes stability and stimulates brain activity.
- **Emotional Fortitude**: Build resilience and strengthen emotional well-being by confronting unresolved emotional issues head-on, and seek professional counsel if you need help with the skills on how to do it. As you grow in resilience,

you stay in a parasympathetic state, which promotes long term health, changes the way your processes, balances hormones, and build energy.

- **Mental Acuity:** Dive deep into personal development and learning in order to improve cognitive function, decision-making, and your perspective on health. You will end up becoming wiser in your decisions.

- **Neurological Clarity:** Address long-standing spinal issues to support autonomic balance, aiding in digestion, sleep, and emotional regulation. As nerve signals strengthen and the body's strength grow, all other functions improve.

Change begins the moment you start applying these principles, but lasting transformation requires consistency and discipline. By committing to these practices, you can unlock your potential, even in adulthood, and create a foundation for long-term health and resilience.

Principles and Actions

We've now completed our guided tour of neurodevelopment, exploring the critical stages from prenatal life through adulthood. Along the way, we've uncovered how challenges at each stage not only disrupt healthy development but also escalate in complexity as children grow older. The longer these issues remain unresolved, the more they compound, creating deeper-rooted problems that can be carried into adulthood. Each stage builds on the one before it, and when structural, chemical, or emotional dysregulation is left unaddressed, the challenges our children face grow increasingly difficult to overcome.

But here's the good news: understanding these patterns equips us with the tools to act. You've learned how the nervous system drives health and development, and now it's time to take that knowledge and put it into practice. We want to ensure you feel empowered, not overwhelmed, with every relevant principle and practical tip you need to support your child's neurodevelopment.

Some steps start at home. These are principles that you can apply at home, which are things you as a parent can take control of through learning, effort, and intentional action. They're foundational steps that require consistency and dedication but are within your power to implement.

Other challenges require professional expertise, things beyond what you can address on your own. This includes clinical interventions that focus on correcting structural, neurological, or other issues that may be interfering with your child's ability to develop and thrive. These interventions, combined with the work you do at home, can dramatically improve your child's quality of life and reduce the stress and strain on their sensitive nervous system.

We've designed the next section of this book to be both actionable, giving you the tools to confidently take the next steps. So, let's begin by focusing on what you can do today.

Chapter 17

At-Home Principles to Apply

Practical Actions Within Your Control

Dr. Ethan

If you've ever tried to raise a child, you know the advice never stops. It comes from everywhere—social media feeds, parenting blogs, family members, church groups, books that contradict each other, and even the occasional stranger at the park. Some of it is helpful, much of it is conflicting, and all of it can feel overwhelming. This chapter isn't about adding to that noise. Instead, it's about focusing on the core principles that actually matter.

Those core principles are captured in the Six Pillars of Health—Mental Acuity, Emotional Fortitude, Chemical Purity, Nutritional Saturation, Structural Stability, and Neurological Clarity. These aren't fads or passing trends; they form the framework through which every action step in this chapter has been filtered. They reflect what neuroscience and developmental research consistently show: that the nervous system thrives when the environment around a child is structured to support calm, balance, and growth. The steps you'll find here are not arbitrary suggestions. They are rooted in an understanding of how the brain wires, repairs, and adapts throughout development—and how daily choices can either strengthen or strain that process. This chapter takes those scientific truths and translates them into practical steps you can use every day.

What follows are actionable ways to bring the Six Pillars to life inside your home. Rather than treating each pillar as a separate checklist, these practices reflect how the pillars overlap and reinforce one another in real-world settings. You don't need to apply everything at once, and perfection isn't the goal. What matters is a steady commitment to principles that have been shown to protect and strengthen neurodevelopment. By using the Six Pillars as your guide, you'll know which habits are worth keeping and which ones to let go—creating an environment where your child's brain and body can grow resilient, adaptable, and healthy for the long run.

Actionable Steps for Parents: Integrating the Six Pillars of Health Across Developmental Stages

Set Priorities Together

One of the most powerful things you can do for your family's health is to treat health as a shared mission, not a solo project. Set aside intentional time—just as you would for a budget meeting or family planning night—for both parents to sit down and evaluate the Six Pillars of Health. Ask simple but revealing questions: Which pillars are strong for us right now? Which ones feel shaky? Where do we see room to grow? This isn't about blame or criticism; it's about alignment. Once you and your spouse have clarity, bring your children into the conversation in an age-appropriate way. Let them see that health is a family priority and invite them into the plan. When kids know the "why" behind your family's habits they're far more likely to embrace those habits as part of the family identity. Unity around your health priorities transforms scattered good intentions into a family culture that consistently builds strong brains and bodies.

Track Developmental Milestones

Just like a growth chart helps you track your child's height and weight, a milestone chart helps you track the progress of their brain and body working together. Regularly refer to a reliable motor milestone chart (see Appendix A) to ensure your child is hitting age-appropriate benchmarks—rolling over, crawling, walking, balancing, and so on. These milestones aren't just cute moments; they're critical signs that the nervous system is wiring correctly. If you notice your child is consistently delayed in meeting these milestones, don't wait and hope they'll "grow out of it." Instead, seek professional guidance from a trusted provider such as your pediatrician, an upper cervical chiropractor, or a pediatric chiropractor. Early recognition and support can make all the difference in keeping your child's neurodevelopment on track.

Reduce Neurologic Stress

Your child's environment is more than just the outside world—it's everything that surrounds them each day, from family rhythms to household habits. This environment has a direct impact on their nervous system and overall development. Take an honest look at the daily atmosphere your child is growing up in: Are routines consistent, or unpredictable? Are screens filling more hours than play and rest? Are parents modeling the same behaviors they ask of their kids? Are siblings treated fairly and consistently? And are there hidden stressors —like processed foods, chemical exposures, or unhealthy substances— that may be weighing on their system? These environmental factors may seem small on their own, but together they create a steady background of either safety and stability, or stress and confusion. By identifying and removing sources of neurologic stress, you give your child's brain the clear, consistent input it needs to grow resilient and strong.

Evaluate Interventions Thoughtfully

When children aren't feeling well, the body often shows it through symptoms like fever, cough, difficulty focusing, or even complaints of pain. It's easy to think of these as the main problem, but in reality they are signals pointing to something deeper that needs attention. Our culture often teaches us to simply cover these symptoms with medication, but that only masks what's really happening. As a parent, your role is to look beyond the surface and recognize what these signals may be indicating, then make informed choices about how to respond. This means equipping yourself with knowledge about both modern interventions—such as medications, vaccines, or procedures—and holistic practices, so you can weigh the benefits and risks with clarity. Avoid making decisions based on quick social media advice or trending hacks. Instead, take the time to investigate, consult trusted professionals, and reflect on how any intervention aligns with your family's health priorities and the Six Pillars framework. Thoughtful evaluation ensures you're not just reacting to symptoms but rather making choices that support long-term brain and body health.

Create Predictable Routines

Children thrive when life follows a rhythm. Predictability calms the nervous system by giving the brain a sense of safety, while inconsistency breeds stress and uncertainty. When a child can anticipate the flow of the day—knowing what comes next and what to expect— their mind can rest, and their body can grow without the hidden tension of unpredictability. This is why routines are not about rigidity but about creating a dependable structure that supports healthy neurodevelopment.

Simple routines anchor a child's day. A consistent morning routine, such as waking at the same time, eating breakfast together, and preparing for the day calmly, sets the tone for steadiness. Bedtime routines—lowering the lights, shutting off screens, reading together, and going to sleep at the same hour—help regulate the circadian rhythm and prepare the brain for restorative rest. Family meals, when shared at regular times and without screens, build connection and emotional security. Chore routines, where children take part in maintaining the home, give them a sense of responsibility and value within the family system.

Beyond the daily rhythm, weekly patterns also matter. A predictable weekend routine with a mix of rest, free play, and intentional family activities gives balance to a child's week. Dedicated one-on-one time between each parent and each child—whether a short drive, a walk, or a simple outing—reinforces belonging and individual attention. Equally important is dedicated one-on-one time between Mom and Dad, going on dates or having dedicated date nights at home, communicates stability at the foundation of the family.

Over time, this sense of safety frees the child's brain to focus on learning and creativity, key elements of neurodevelopment. Predictable routines become more than schedules; they are the invisible framework that allows children to flourish.

Model Healthy Emotional Responses

Children learn emotional regulation from their parents—not so much from what their parents *say*, but from what their parents *do*. A common mistake is adopting a "do as I say, not as I do" approach, but children almost always imitate what they observe. A more effective model is, *"Do as I say, because I do as I say."* When parents show steadiness in the midst of stress, they're giving their child a living example of how to handle challenges. Over time, this example helps the child's nervous system remain calmer and more adaptable, even when life feels overwhelming.

That's why it can be helpful to let children see constructive responses in real time. If frustration rises in traffic, for instance, a parent might say aloud, "I feel irritated right now, but since I can't control traffic, I'm going to take a deep breath and put on some music while we wait." Or when tackling a hard project at home, they might invite their child to watch them work through it patiently, showing that difficult things can be handled without losing control. These moments give children both a picture and a pathway for emotional stability.

Modeling also includes forgiveness and reconciliation. If a parent reacts sharply, it can be powerful to come back to the child and say, "That response wasn't the way I wanted to handle it. I'm sorry—will you forgive me? I love you." This not only repairs the relationship but also shows the child that mistakes don't have to lead to lingering conflict. Without this modeling, children may learn to bottle up frustration or hold onto bitterness, patterns that add unnecessary stress to both the body and nervous system over time.

Choose Mentors and Role Models Carefully

Remember the saying, "It takes a village to raise a child"? That village needs to be carefully chosen. A supportive environment provides your child with a network of trusted adults who align with your family's values and health goals. These mentors don't just shape behavior; they also help regulate a child's nervous system. When children know they are surrounded by consistent, caring adults, their brains register safety, which lowers stress responses and frees up energy for growth, learning, and creativity.

Children build pathways by mirroring what they observe. Adults who live with courage, wisdom, discipline, and compassion give the nervous system repeated patterns of stability and integrity to copy. These mentors also provide trusted voices when your child has questions you may not be able to answer yourself. And when those voices come from individuals who are raising their own families with purpose, your child sees what a life of consistency looks like in practice.

You might connect your child with a coach who emphasizes character over trophies, a teacher who sparks curiosity, a family friend who demonstrates kindness and hospitality, or a church leader who models humility. These examples create "reference points" for your child's brain, reinforcing the same values from multiple angles. Over time, that consistent reinforcement strengthens both neural pathways and character development. A carefully built village doesn't replace your role as a parent—it expands the sources of safety, perspective, and encouragement in your child's life. And neurologically, a child who feels supported by a strong network of honorable influences is far more likely to meet life's challenges with resilience and confidence.

Eliminate Harmful Chemical Exposures

A child's developing brain and nervous system are especially sensitive to the environment. What they breathe, touch, and drink affects the efficiency at which their brain and body communicate. When communication pathways are overloaded with toxins from artificial food ingredients, synthetic cleaners, impure air or water, the nervous system works harder than it should, trying to mitigate damage caused by those toxins. This results in your child having less energy for healthy growth and development. That's why being mindful of your child's daily exposures can go a long way in supporting calm, balanced neurodevelopment.

Household cleaners are one of the simplest places to start. Many contain harsh chemicals—like ammonia, chlorine, phthalates, or formaldehyde—that have been linked to hormone disruption, respiratory issues, and developmental concerns. Since children breathe more quickly than adults and absorb more through their skin, they're especially vulnerable. Choosing gentler, more naturally based alternatives, such as vinegar and baking soda, removes unnecessary stress from their system while still keeping the home clean.

Air and water also matter. The brain depends on a steady supply of oxygen to function at its best, and poor air quality can interfere with focus, sleep, and long-term neurological health. Opening windows for fresh airflow, using a high-quality purifier in your child's bedroom, or adding air-filtering plants—such as snake plants, peace lilies, spider plants, or bamboo palms—can noticeably improve the quality of the air they breathe. Similarly, using a reliable water filter ensures fewer chemicals enter their system daily. Clean water and clean air may sound simple, but they are two of the most powerful supports you can provide for the nervous system.

The goal isn't to create a bubble—it's to reduce the invisible background stressors that quietly tax the brain. When the load is lighter, your child's nervous system has more freedom to do what it was designed to do: grow, adapt, and thrive.

Eliminate Harmful Screen and Media Exposures

Technology and media can be just as taxing on a child's developing brain as chemical exposures in the environment. Excessive screen time overstimulates the brain's dopamine system, training children to crave constant novelty and instant gratification. This kind of stimulation rewires attention, making it harder to focus, imagine, and self-regulate. A child's nervous system thrives on rhythm and balance, but screens often pull them into a state of hyperarousal that leaves the brain restless and unsettled.

What children watch and hear matters as much as how much time they spend on screens. Just because a movie, book, or song feels nostalgic to you doesn't mean it is appropriate for your child at their stage of development. Take the example of *The Lion King*: while beloved by many, the scene where Simba watches his father die can stir feelings of abandonment in a young child who otherwise feels secure. These moments aren't automatically harmful, but they do require follow-up. Taking a few minutes afterward to talk through the emotions helps a child process the experience in a healthy way. This turns potentially overwhelming moments into opportunities for growth, giving the nervous system practice in digesting complex feelings.

The same principle applies to music. Songs from your own childhood may carry fond memories, but a closer listen often reveals lyrics that are vulgar, violent, or dismissive of the values you want to cultivate. Just because something is nostalgic doesn't mean it's appropriate. Children's brains are constantly wiring themselves around what they see and hear, and repeated exposure to unhealthy messages can subtly shape how they think, feel, and act.

Being thoughtful about media isn't about sheltering your child from the world; it's about giving their nervous system the right kind of input to mature at the pace it's ready for. When parents guide both the *amount* and the *type* of media their children consume they give their child's brain the best chance to be thoughtful, focused, and attentive.

Choose More Whole Foods (and Read Labels Carefully)

Food is one of the most powerful tools for shaping your child's brain and body. The closer it is to its natural form, the better it fuels healthy neurodevelopment. Fresh fruits, vegetables, high-quality proteins, and nutrient-dense fats give the nervous system the building blocks it needs to grow, repair, and regulate. A simple principle is to eat what's in season—this naturally varies your child's diet across the year, providing a wide range of vitamins and minerals that support brain growth. Rotating proteins is also helpful: lighter options like chicken balance well with fattier cuts of beef or pork, which provide essential fat-soluble nutrients. Foods rich in probiotics, such as yogurt, kefir, kimchi, or pickled vegetables, further support gut health—often called the "second brain"—which plays a direct role in nutrient absorption and neurological stability.

It also helps to remember that carbohydrates, proteins, and fats are not inherently bad. These macronutrients each play essential roles in the body and brain. The brain relies heavily on carbohydrates, best consumed from fruits and vegetables where natural fiber prevents sugar overload. Proteins supply the building blocks for hormones and tissue repair. Fats act as carriers, transporting nutrients and stabilizing cells. In the right proportions, all three support balanced development. As a general guide your child should eat the following proportions of each macronutrient each day:

- **Proteins:** 1–1.5 grams per kilogram ($\approx$ 0.45–0.7 grams per pound)
- **Carbohydrates:** ~2 grams per kilogram ($\approx$ 0.9 grams per pound)
- **Fats:** 0.5–1 gram per kilogram of body weight ($\approx$ 0.2–0.45 grams per pound)

Helping your child meet these daily nutritional goals gives their body the fuel its needs for physical and neurological development. Understanding these ranges can help explain why your child's appetite changes from day to day and meal to meal. If a child has not gotten the right balance of macronutrients at a meal, they might feel hungry sooner. But if they've had a meal that was rich in macronutrients they may not feel as hungry for the next meal. This is because your child's brain knows when the body needs more of a certain nutrient. You don't have to force your child to hit these numbers every day but consistently providing your child with meals complete with balanced fats, proteins, and carbohydrates will lead to a filled belly, happy demeanor, and proper nutritional saturation.

When packaged foods do find their way into your home, it's worth taking a moment to read the labels. Additives like artificial sweeteners (aspartame, sucralose, sorbitol) can disrupt the gut microbiome, while preservatives such as nitrates and nitrites (commonly found in processed meats) have been linked to long-term health risks. Food dyes like Red 40 have even been associated with worsening ADHD and other developmental challenges. Since the gut and brain are so closely linked, anything that irritates digestion can also disrupt neurological health. A simple rule of thumb is this: if the label looks more like a chemistry set than a food, it's probably not the best fuel for a developing brain.

By focusing on whole, nourishing foods and keeping an eye on the quality of what goes into your child's body, you give their nervous system the raw materials it needs to grow strong, resilient, and clear.

Encourage Regular, Balanced Meals

Children need consistent rhythms around food, just like they do around sleep. Establish clear mealtimes and snack times, and avoid letting eating become an all-day, on-demand event. This not only supports healthy metabolism but also trains your child to listen to true hunger cues instead of constant grazing, which can lead to obesity and emotional eating. Parents often worry if a child doesn't eat as much at one sitting, but remember: if you consistently provide balanced meals at set times, your child won't allow themselves to go hungry.

Introduce variety regularly—rotate proteins, swap out snack types, and bring in new fruits and vegetables. The key is gentle consistency: structured mealtimes paired with steady encouragement to try new foods creates peace for the parent and healthy habits for the child.

Supplement When Necessary

Even the best diets sometimes need extra support. Modern farming practices have depleted soils of key nutrients, leaving fruits and vegetables with less of the vitamins and minerals they once contained. One example is magnesium—a micronutrient essential for metabolic processes, energy production, and sleep regulation. Today, even with a diet rich in produce, many children (and parents) fall short of magnesium's daily requirements. In these cases, supplementation can be an important tool.

Work with a trusted healthcare provider to evaluate your child's nutritional status and identify true deficiencies. Supplementation should never be a shot in the dark; it should fill gaps where the diet alone cannot keep up. When used appropriately, supplements provide the "missing puzzle pieces" to ensure your child's body and brain have everything they need to develop optimally.

Just Play

One of the most important foundations for a child's brain and body is physical play. Movement doesn't just build muscles—it wires the brain. Every jump, climb, balance, or roll creates and strengthens neural pathways that support coordination, focus, and long-term resilience. Unfortunately, many schools are reducing physical activity in favor of extended classroom time, leaving children without the movement their brains and bodies desperately need. That's why it falls to parents to ensure their children have opportunities for daily physical play.

The best movement for young children is full-body activity. Sports and practices that require coordination across the entire body—like gymnastics, martial arts, swimming, dance, or even obstacle-course style training—help build broad motor skills that the brain can use for a lifetime. These kinds of activities also prevent overuse injuries that come from early hyper-specialization in a single sport. Children who play only one sport year-round may develop highly specific movement patterns but lack the broader coordination and injury protection mechanisms that come from variety. In contrast, kids who climb trees, ride bikes, swim, or run through an open field build adaptable skills that carry into adulthood.

Strength training also plays an important role. While children should first master control of their own body weight—running, climbing, crawling, hanging, and balancing—they should eventually learn to lift heavier objects safely. Carrying groceries, moving furniture under supervision, or using age-appropriate weights helps strengthen muscles, bones, and connective tissues. This not only builds immediate resilience but also lays the groundwork for strong bone density and reduced risk of degenerative conditions later in life. In fact, research shows that a lifetime of physical activity is one of the most powerful protectors against Alzheimer's and other cognitive declines in old age. The earlier a physically active lifestyle begins, the longer the brain remains primed for health.

Parents should adopt these same principles for themselves as well. Children who see Mom and Dad active, strong, and playful are far more likely to imitate those habits. The message becomes clear: movement is not just something children are "made" to do—it's a way of life for the whole family.

Teach Proper Posture

When the structures of the spine (muscles, ligaments, fascia, and bones) are upright, coordinated, and balanced, with weight dispersed evenly, physical stresses are absorbed, and the body remains adaptable. Without that balance, even small strains can create long-term problems.

Instead of having to constantly remind your child to "sit up straight," give them a simple mental cue: *pretend there's a ball balancing on top of your head.* If they lean too far forward or too far back, the ball will "roll off." This image helps children naturally elongate their spine and stack their head, shoulders, and hips in proper alignment without constant external correction. Over time, this habit becomes second nature.

If your child struggles to maintain posture because of general weakness, the solution is strength. Encourage play and activities that build core and back strength—climbing, crawling, hanging, or age-appropriate resistance training. But if posture problems persist despite strength-building, the issue may not be muscular at all—it may be neurologic. In these cases, restoring proper brain-body communication is essential, which is the role of an upper cervical chiropractor. By correcting misalignments at the top of the spine, the nervous system can reconnect, allowing posture to improve naturally rather than through constant forced reminders.

Build Healthy Sleep Habits

Sleep is when the body repairs and the brain organizes. During deep rest, your child's nervous system integrates the physical lessons learned during the day and stores new memories for long-term use. Without restorative sleep, both brain and body are left under-recovered. That's why creating strong sleep habits is just as important as nutrition and physical activity.

Start by building a pre-bed routine. About an hour before sleep, dim the lights in the house and turn off screens. Blue light from TVs, tablets, and phones disrupts melatonin production, the hormone that helps the brain shift into sleep. Calming activities like reading together, listening to quiet music, or playing a gentle board game help downshift the nervous system and prepare the body for rest.

The sleep environment matters as much as the routine. A cooler room—ideally around 65°F, or at least with a fan running—supports deeper sleep and more restorative rest. Keep the room as dark as possible to avoid stimulating the brain. A firm but comfortable mattress gives stable support, and pillows should hold the neck in a neutral position: on the back, supporting the natural cervical curve, or on the side, filling the space between shoulder and head. Stomach-sleeping should be avoided, as it twists the neck and strains the still-developing spine. Using a thin lightweight blanket can even increase comfort without overheating your child. For infants less than 1 year old, skip pillows and blankets entirely until they are old enough to safely move objects away from their airway, to reduce the risk of SIDS (Sudden Infant Death Syndrome). Instead of blankets, use swaddles (used until your baby can roll from back to belly), sleep sacks or footy-pajamas to keep the baby warm.

Consistency is the key that ties it all together. A regular bedtime and wake time regulate your child's circadian rhythm, training the body to anticipate rest and energy at the right times. Whenever possible, sync this rhythm with the natural rise and fall of the sun. Daily physical activity also makes sleep more effective—when the body has used energy throughout the day, rest becomes both deeper and easier to achieve. Finally, in the morning, avoid starting the day with screens. Giving the brain a chance to wake naturally allows the nervous system to rise gradually into alertness instead of being shocked into hyperstimulation.

Strong sleep habits don't just give your child energy for the next day—they rebuild the body, solidify learning, and strengthen the brain's long-term resilience.

Strengthening the Nervous System

Everything we've discussed—nutrition, movement, sleep, posture, emotional resilience, and environmental health—ultimately supports one central system: the nervous system. A balanced nervous system shifts naturally between the "fight-or-flight" state (sympathetic) and the "rest-and-digest" state (parasympathetic). Both are vital: healing and learning happen in the parasympathetic state, while strength and exertion require sympathetic activation. Training the body to move smoothly between these states is key for healthy development. Parents can support this balance in a few practical ways:

Teaching your child to breathe with their nose rather than their mouth and with their diaphragm rather than their shoulders. A simple exercise is to place a stuffed animal on their stomach and have them watch it rise and fall as they breathe through their nose. Nose breathing goes hand-in-hand with this, helping filter and warm the air while ensuring better oxygen exchange. If your child cannot breathe comfortably through their nose, consider consulting a myofunctional therapist, an orthodontist, or airway specialist for evaluation.

Prioritize Chiropractic Care for Maintenance

Many children do not need intensive neurologic intervention but rather preventative care. This means that consistent care with an upper cervical or pediatric chiropractor helps ensure there is no interference between the brain and body at the most critical level—the brainstem. With clear communication, the nervous system can adapt more easily to the ever-growing stressors surrounding today's children (physical injuries, infections, family stress, peer-related stress, stress from increasing responsibilities). A well-maintained and more adaptable nervous system means when your child encounters these stressors, they have a better opportunity for speedy recovery with limited to no lingering effects.

Combined with the healthy habits outlined earlier in this chapter, chiropractic care further supports a nervous system that is stable, resilient, and able to fuel a stronger, healthier brain and body.

Sometimes It Gets Clinical

While it might feel overwhelming, the key to reinforcing your child's nervous system is thoughtful, consistent action. The sections above are not all-encompassing, but it should give you a good jumping off point. Start where you are, grow in understanding, and adapt these principles to your child's unique needs. The actions above, rooted in an understanding of the principles within the Six Pillars, provide a foundation for fostering optimal neurodevelopment and creating a healthy environment where your child can thrive—today and for a lifetime.

Still, even the most dedicated parents may reach a point where at-home strategies aren't enough on their own. That's when having professional support becomes invaluable. In the next chapter, we'll look at how specialized clinical care can work alongside the principles you're already practicing bringing even greater clarity and balance to your child's nervous system.

Chapter 18

Clinical Help for Your Kids

How To Restore Lost Function

Dr. Ethan

I came home from class to find my wife preparing a snack for our daughter. She seemed unusually elated for someone just making a snack.

After setting my things down, I scooped up my daughter, covering her in a big hug and kiss. She promptly pulled away, wriggling in protest —Daddy had rudely interrupted her snack.

That's when I caught it—the unmistakable aroma of freshly baked dinner rolls drifting through the air.

"Those smell amazing, love!" I said as I moved to greet my wife, who, despite handling a newly turned one-year-old all day, still looked as lovely as ever.

"Thanks, baby," she replied, planting a quick peck on my lips. Then, with a knowing smile, she added, "They aren't the only buns in the oven either."

Her words hit me mid-thought. *Not the only buns in the ove—*

My eyes widened. "Wait... what!? Are we having another baby!?"

"Yup," she said, beaming.

I let out a breathless laugh, my excitement mirrored in her eyes. Amid the happy squeals of our firstborn, we embraced the incredible blessing of another child. Thank God for this chance to grow our family.

As the pregnancy progressed, my wife continued her chiropractic care, maintained her massage therapy work, exercised regularly, and remained an incredible wife and mother.

At the 20-week anatomy scan, we decided to find out if our daughter would be getting a little brother or sister. Sitting in the ultrasound room, we watched the screen with bated breath as the technician moved the probe over my wife's belly.

Then, BOOM—there was no mistaking it. Our baby boy made the announcement for us in the clearest way possible.

The room filled with laughter.

"There you have it, Mom and Dad," the technician chuckled, composing herself. "It's a boy!"

We basked in the excitement, celebrating our son-to-be. But as the scan continued, the technician's demeanor shifted. Her tone became more professional, almost somber.

"Okay, parents, we have two things to look at." She pointed to a bright white mark on the screen. "This is what we call a 'soft sign.' It doesn't indicate with 100% certainty a developmental issue, but it can be linked to one. This one here"—she pointed again—"and this one"—another spot we hadn't noticed—"are markers associated with Trisomy 18 and 21. Nothing to be overly concerned about, but we'll need to inform your OB so she can guide you on the next steps."

We thanked her and the rest of the team, walking out of the office trying to mask the sinking feeling in our hearts.

"Nothing to be concerned about."

That did nothing to calm us.

We turned to research. We knew the body was capable of healing. We had no family history of either condition, and we understood that genetics alone weren't the whole picture. Development required an epigenetic component—the activation of specific genes at specific times, influenced by the environment. If something had triggered those markers, we believed it could also be reversed.

Everything we initially found said these markers were genetic, set in stone. But we decided to change the question. Instead of searching for *causes* of Trisomy 18 and 21, we asked, *What environmental factors contribute to genetic instability?*

That new perspective led us to information on genetic mutations linked to excessive processed food consumption, both during pregnancy and before conception. We found evidence that chemically toxic food dyes were associated with genetic disorders and neurodevelopmental issues.

We had always loved gummy bears—but those food dyes had to go. So did all chemically toxic "foods."

We overhauled our diet, eliminating everything artificial and ensuring we consumed only whole, nourishing foods. We were committed.

At the next scan, the markers were gone.

Our little boy was back on track.

As the due date approached, we felt ready. We had endured the stress of genetic scares and balanced my school responsibilities with my wife's work, but now we were prepared for the most natural birth possible.

Breathwork was practiced, affirmations were prepared, go-bags were packed. In just two weeks, we would finally meet our son.

Then, one afternoon, my wife called me in the middle of the day— something she never did.

Her voice was shaky, close to tears. *The hospital had called.*

"They said they're ready for my induction," she choked out.

I frowned. "What induction? We didn't schedule an induction."

"I don't know," she said, her voice breaking. "Do we have to go? I don't want to be induced!"

She was overwhelmed, crying, hyperventilating. She knew her stress was affecting the baby, which only made her stress worse.

It had never occurred to me that we might be expected to keep an appointment we never made.

After calming her down, we talked it through and made a decision. My wife called the hospital back.

"We are not coming in for an induction. We will have the baby naturally."

Concerned, our OB called to warn us about potential complications if labor became too difficult.

"Have any of your patients been under consistent chiropractic care through pregnancy?" I asked.

A pause. "...No."

"We trust my wife's body. We'll wait, and our baby will come at the right time."

That was the end of it. A week later, labor began.

We made a calm but urgent drive to the hospital, fully prepared for this moment. The night team respected our birth plan, ensuring everything progressed naturally. Even our previously concerned OB entered the room with excitement—our baby was coming!

As my wife gave one final push, our son's pink head emerged, and the doctor reached to catch him. But in the rush of the moment, his tiny head bent sharply to the side.

Something was wrong.

Our daughter had cried immediately at birth, latched effortlessly, and had been alert and responsive. This time was different.

Our son wasn't crying. He wasn't really moving. His pink color faded to blue.

A chill ran through me. *Where was the life in my son?*

The urgency in the room escalated. The birth team jumped into action. "He's okay. He'll cry, he'll latch, he'll be fine," they reassured us. But he wasn't.

He wasn't crying.

He wasn't latching.

My wife, desperate, pleaded with him: "C'mon, buddy, cry for us. You can do it."

Her tear-filled eyes met mine. *Do something.*

Then, I heard it in my head: You can do this. You're trained for this.

I had prepared for this exact moment. With my hands moving quickly yet precisely, I analyzed his tiny frame. After I gently adjusted his upper neck, his nerve function was restored.

In an instant, his pink color returned.

Then, a deep inhale—

And a bellowing cry and a quick latch.

Relief washed over us as he turned and latched onto his mama, his little body full of life again. Our son's nervous system was restored. His health—his very future—had been given back to him in that moment.

Welcome to the world, Eli Amadeus Surprenant.

Conviction Under Pressure

The strength of a person's resolve is always tested under pressure. Moments like the one we experienced with our son have tested us time and time again. The world will tell you to take the easy path, to follow the conventional way, but those are the moments when your convictions—what you *know* to be true—face the ultimate test.

Would we ever put our children in danger just to prove a point? Of course not. Everything we teach, everything we recommend, and everything we do clinically begins with our own families first—applied in the moments that matter most, even when the stakes are life and death.

The recommendations we make are not based on fear of punishment by a medical board or the pressure to conform to mainstream expectations. We teach what we teach, and we make the recommendations we make, because this is how the body is *designed* to function.

With that in mind, we encourage you to take everything we share with the seriousness it deserves. The decisions you make for your children matter. They shape not only their immediate health but also their long-term well-being.

Systematic Approach

Dr. Chris

When things aren't going as expected, and the problems seem beyond your understanding, it's critical to seek the right kind of professional help. This chapter provides specific guidance on how to pursue professional intervention when at-home principles aren't enough. These strategies include both preventative measures and intervention solutions.

Dr. Ethan and I follow a clear, sequenced approach when assessing the health of our own children. If something seems off—whether it's difficulty sleeping, eating, digesting, or frequent illness—our first step is to check their nervous system. Unless there is obvious trauma, such as bleeding or a fracture, we prioritize assessing the brain-body connection to ensure clear communication within the nervous system.

Why? Because every function in the body depends on the nervous system for coordination and regulation—from muscle movements to digestion to emotional responses. If that communication is disrupted, the body cannot function as it should.

And when the nervous system does not function properly, there are clear symptoms throughout the various stages of neurodevelopment that indicate dysfunction. Some of the more common symptoms we've already discussed include:

- **Infancy:** Difficulty latching, colic, torticollis, or infrequent pooping.
- **Toddlerhood:** Delayed speech, sleep issues, balance problems, or frequent infections.
- **Early Childhood:** Chronic fatigue, emotional dysregulation, or social withdrawal.
- **Grade School Years:** Difficulty focusing, posture problems, scoliosis, academic struggles, and persistent illness.
- **Teenage Years:** Exhaustion, emotional instability, or signs of depression.

We've mentioned it throughout the book, but the approach we use to correct nervous system dysfunction is called Upper Cervical Care.

This differs significantly from general chiropractic care, which often involves full-spine adjustments and manual manipulation. Upper Cervical Care is highly specialized, focusing exclusively on the upper cervical spine, particularly the atlas (C1) and axis (C2) vertebrae. These two bones play a pivotal role in housing and protecting the brainstem, which regulates nearly every automatic function in the body.

The Advanced Orthogonal Technique

There are several Upper Cervical adjusting methods designed to correct misalignments in the upper neck. Some approaches involve manual adjustments, while others utilize precision instruments. Regardless of the method, the goal remains the same: to restore proper alignment and stabilize the upper cervical spine, allowing the nervous system to function optimally and communicate effectively along its delicate nerve pathways.

In our practice, we use a highly specialized Upper Cervical technique called the Advanced Orthogonal Technique. This method uses a percussive sound wave instrument to shift the misaligned vertebrae without physically touching the skin. The adjustment comes from a table-mounted mechanism that delivers a controlled sonic impulse, ensuring maximum precision, consistency, and safety.

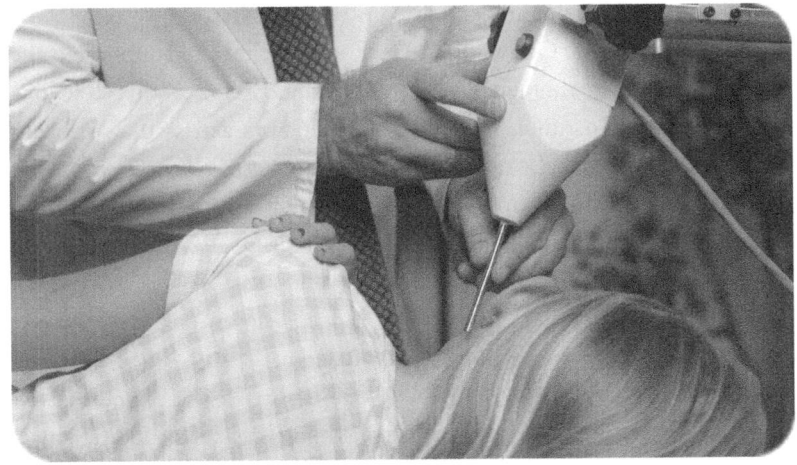

The instrument's stylus is positioned just off the skin, and inside the mechanism, a solenoid generates a carefully calibrated percussive wave that targets the atlas (C1) vertebra. This precise force gently shifts the misaligned bone back into its proper position without any twisting, cracking, or popping of the neck.

To help illustrate how this works, consider how sound is actually force traveling through air. Imagine you're sitting at a stoplight, and a car pulls up beside you with booming bass speakers. You not only hear the music—you feel the vibrations pass through your car and into your body. This happens because sound waves carry energy through the air and surrounding materials and transfer that energy to you. Similarly, ocean waves carry energy through water—when they crash onto shore, it's not just the water hitting you; it's the transfer of energy from the wave into your body that you feel.

The Advanced Orthogonal Technique harnesses this same principle—using the percussive force within a sound wave to realign the atlas without the need for physical pressure or manipulation.

To ensure precision, we take detailed imaging before making any adjustments. These images allow us to accurately assess the shapes, positions, and misalignments of the upper cervical vertebrae. By carefully measuring these images, we calculate exact vectors—specific angles and force directions—to customize each child's correction with the utmost precision. This individualized care plan ensures the best results while prioritizing the child's comfort and safety.

The Advanced Orthogonal Institute teaches and upholds the standards of this technique. As of this writing, I serve as the Executive Director of the Institute, where we train doctors across the nation in this method. We are also affiliated with the International Chiropractic Association's Council on Upper Cervical Care, an organization dedicated to maintaining high standards of care, advancing research, and continually improving best practices in Upper Cervical work. This collaboration among our Upper Cervical colleagues ensures that our standards remain at the cutting edge of healthcare.

The Advanced Orthogonal Technique is suitable for patients of all ages, but for children over six, their developing skeletal structure allows us to apply the same precision-based approach as we do for adults. By this age, their bones have begun to take on a more defined shape and density, making it possible to obtain clear imaging and precise vector calculations to guide corrections. This ensures that we can realign the spine with the highest degree of accuracy, helping to restore proper neurological function and stability.

However, for children under six, there are important considerations due to their ongoing skeletal development. Their bones are still forming, and their upper cervical spine has a more simplified joint structure, which requires a modified approach to ensure both safety and effectiveness.

Modifications for Children Under Six

While the Advanced Orthogonal Technique is highly effective for all ages, caring for young children requires adaptations tailored to their developmental stage. Because their bones are still soft and their joint structures are more flexible, we typically do not take x-rays unless there are clear neurological concerns that warrant further investigation.

Some of the conditions that may require imaging for children under six include:

- Airway problems that interfere with breathing.
- Severe balance issues affecting mobility and coordination.
- Torticollis, where the head tilts and the neck muscles tighten abnormally.
- Seizures or fainting episodes which may indicate brainstem involvement.

For the majority of young children, a thorough physical and neurological examination is sufficient to assess alignment and determine the best course of care. Adjustments are performed using gentle, low-force techniques, either with a light hand adjustment or a small, instrument-assisted tap, ensuring safety, comfort, and precision. The goal remains the same: to restore proper upper cervical alignment and support optimal neurodevelopment, helping the nervous system function without interference.

This modified approach enables even the youngest patients, including newborns, to benefit from Upper Cervical Care, promoting optimal neurological function from the very start of life.

Other Clinical Care for Your Child

While Upper Cervical Care is central to laying the foundation for healthy neurodevelopment and restoring neurological clarity in children, it is not the only solution for every issue. Some children face challenges stemming from chemical toxicity, nutritional deficiencies, or more significant structural and developmental issues. Because of this, a comprehensive and multidisciplinary approach is often necessary.

However, finding the right kind of providers isn't just about credentials or the letters after a doctor's name—it's about their approach to care. The best doctors aren't necessarily the most credentialed but rather the ones who think in a certain way. If your goal is to restore your child's health, rather than just mask symptoms, then you need to seek out professionals who focus on root causes.

When looking for clinical support for your child, prioritize professionals who follow these three essential principles:

1. A Root Cause Focus

Seek professionals who identify and address the root cause of your child's health challenges rather than just managing symptoms. True healing comes from restoring function, not suppressing warning signs. If a doctor's primary focus is symptom management, their approach will more than likely be reactive rather than restorative.

2. A Restorative and Holistic Approach

Prioritize care providers who work with the body's natural processes, aiming to restore self-regulation rather than override it. In general, this means a more holistic approach—one that considers how different systems of the body interact.

Unfortunately, holistic care has been dismissed or misunderstood by many, but at its core, it simply means restoring the body's ability to function as it was designed. If a child is nutritionally deficient, then working with a specialist who focuses on gut health, proper nutrient intake, and guiding parents in restructuring home nutrition is the best course of action. On the other hand, if a child breaks a leg, the immediate and necessary action would be to visit the emergency room or an orthopedic specialist.

The point is that both approaches have their place. The key difference is that holistic care works to restore self-regulation, while intervention-based care is necessary for acute injuries or crises. A healthy balance between the two is critical for comprehensive healthcare.

3. Specialized Expertise

When dealing with complex health issues, working with specialists —rather than generalists—is often necessary. A jack-of-all-trades approach can miss the mark, whereas a specialist pinpoints the root cause and provides targeted solutions.

Many highly specialized providers also tend to be more collaborative because their focus isn't on competing in the marketplace —it's on solving the problems they've spent years studying. Specialists dedicate their careers to deep expertise, ensuring they have the right tools and resources to truly restore function in the children they help.

To assist parents in finding the right professionals, we've compiled a list of specialists in Appendix B. These types of providers include:
- Airway Orthodontists
- Craniosacral Therapists
- Functional Medicine Practitioners
- And more…

This reference list can help parents identify the right care for their child's specific needs.

Bringing It All Together

Whether through Upper Cervical Care, nutritional therapy, airway development, or other clinical interventions, the ultimate goal remains the same: to work with the body's natural processes to restore function and balance.

By seeking out root cause-focused professionals who understand how to support healthy neurodevelopment, parents can equip their children with the tools they need to grow, thrive, and reach their full potential.

However, no intervention, treatment, or professional guidance can replace the power of parental influence. You can apply at-home principles, seek clinical support, and provide access to the best possible resources, but the greatest impact on your child's lifelong health is you —the example you set, the habits you model, and the way you prioritize your own well-being.

Chapter 19

Parents, It Starts With You

Build a Legacy of Health

Dr. Ethan

As parents, we all dream of giving our children the best possible start in life—hoping they'll grow up healthier, stronger, and wiser than we ever were. But here's a truth that can't be ignored: your child's definition of health is shaped by your example. They are constantly watching, learning, and imitating. You are their most consistent role model.

Your health, relationships, habits, fitness, nutrition, structure, and care for your own nervous system shape what your child perceives as "normal." Whether consciously or subconsciously, they will measure their own behaviors and decisions against the example you set. If you say one thing about health but live another way, children notice the inconsistency—and it can lead them to adopt unhealthy patterns themselves. The strongest way to influence your child's future health is to lead with action. By caring for your own well-being first, you provide them with a living model of the habits and resilience you hope they will carry into their own lives.

Parents Set the Home Standard

It is your responsibility to define what health looks like in your home—not just for your children, but for the entire family. This isn't about achieving perfection; it's about setting a clear standard and striving for intentional, consistent growth. By working daily to improve your own health by just 1%, you model the pursuit of progress, resilience, and self-discipline. And because your children are starting younger—learning from your example—their ability to grow and adapt will far exceed yours over the course of their lifetime.

First, ask yourself: *How can I become 1% better for my child today?* When you find your own points of improvement and act on them, you are modeling the behaviors your family can emulate. Demonstrating the health standards you set—by eating quality foods, prioritizing movement, maintaining strength, detoxing your environment, and caring for your nervous system—creates a living example of what health looks like in practice.

From there, you can lead your family in practical steps that establish the culture and environment of your home. Set goals together, just as we discussed earlier, by creating specific family health goals such as eating more home-cooked meals, drinking more water, doing a challenging physical activity, or reducing screen time. Be honest about challenges and acknowledge when you fall short, modeling resilience by getting back on track. Celebrate progress, not perfection, recognizing small wins like completing a family hike or trying a new recipe, and emphasize effort and growth over unrealistic ideals. Finally, commit to lifelong learning by showing your children that health is an ongoing journey—whether through reading a new book, trying a new exercise, or experimenting with better nutrition.

Freedom Within Limits

Setting the standard also requires establishing boundaries. Boundaries are not restrictive—they are empowering. They give children a sense of security, allowing them to explore, grow, and develop within a safe framework.

A fascinating study from 2006 illustrates this concept well. Researchers observed preschool children in two different playground environments. In the first, there was no fence—the children hesitated to venture far from their teacher, staying close for security. In the second, a fence defined the playground's boundaries. The children played without hesitation throughout the entire playground environment, even far from their teacher. Here, the children felt free to explore and play with confidence, knowing they were safe within the set limits.

The conclusion was clear: boundaries create freedom. Far from restricting growth, clearly defined limits allow children to understand expectations, feel secure, and develop independence. They also reduce stress by giving the nervous system predictability and structure, helping children focus on learning, playing, and thriving.

Boundaries also foster autonomy. Within safe limits, children can take risks, make decisions, and develop confidence in their ability to navigate the world. Moreover, boundaries guide without micromanagement, allowing kids to learn through experience while knowing they are supported.

Here is a simple action plan that helps you establish healthy home boundaries:

- **Define the "Fence" Together** – Explain family rules in a way your child understands. Be mindful of what truly matters —like limiting front yard play for safety, but letting them get messy in the dirt.
- **Model Respect for Boundaries** – Show your child that you also follow rules—whether it's respecting family agreements, maintaining work-life balance, or prioritizing self-care.
- **Be Consistent** – Inconsistency (between parents or within different settings) confuses children and weakens boundaries. Stick to the limits you set, even when inconvenient.
- **Allow Freedom Within Limits** – Once boundaries are in place, let your child explore freely within them. Give them space to make choices and learn from the outcomes.
- **Adjust as Needed** – As your child grows, adapt boundaries to match their developmental stage. A toddler's limits will be

different from a teenager's, but the principle remains the same.

A Legacy of Health, Resilience, and Neurological Clarity

Investing in your health and setting clear boundaries isn't just about building good habits—it's about creating an environment where your family's nervous systems can function at their best. A well-regulated nervous system is the command center for all growth, emotional stability, and resilience. When you prioritize your own health, you model the stability and clarity that will anchor your family through life's challenges.

The daily choices you make—nourishing your body, prioritizing movement, reducing stress, and creating structure—directly impact not just your own well-being but your child's ability to thrive. By committing to these principles, you break cycles of poor health and redefine what it means for your family to flourish.

Too often, parents are taught to manage surface-level symptoms rather than uncover what is happening beneath them. If a child struggles with sleep, the recommended solution might be melatonin. If they face repeated infections, another round of antibiotics is prescribed. If attention falters, stimulant medication is recommended. While each of these approaches may provide temporary relief, they rarely address the root cause—the underlying stress or dysregulation in the nervous system that is driving the struggle in the first place.

When you as a parent begin to look deeper, you change the trajectory not only for yourself but for your children. Instead of asking, "How do I quiet this symptom?" the better question becomes, "Why is the symptom here at all?" By seeking to understand the root—whether structural misalignments, chronic stress patterns, nutritional imbalances, or toxic exposures—you uncover the real drivers of dysfunction. This approach doesn't just quiet the noise of symptoms; it restores clarity to the system so the body can function the way it was designed.

Root-cause thinking is one of the greatest legacies you can pass down to your children. It models a way of viewing health that is proactive, not reactive—one that builds resilience instead of dependency. By showing your children that real healing comes from addressing causes, not covering symptoms, you give them the tools to navigate life with confidence, clarity, and hope for lasting health.

Boundaries support this same process by giving your child predictability and structure. Just as a fenced playground allows freedom within limits, the clear standards you set at home create security and space for growth.

Ultimately, every one of the Six Pillars of Health—Mental Acuity, Emotional Fortitude, Chemical Purity, Nutritional Saturation, Structural Stability, and Neurological Clarity—exists to strengthen and protect the nervous system. Stewarding these pillars while seeking root causes of dysfunction ensures that your child's body and brain are set up to thrive.

As parents, your commitment to these principles creates more than habits—it creates a legacy. By leading with clarity and purpose, you not only shape your child's future but also lay the foundation for generations to come.

Appendix A

Early Developmental Milestones Checklist

A Proper Order for Proper Development

This appendix outlines the key developmental milestones that children are expected to reach at various ages. These checkpoints reflect both physical and neurological growth, though most of the listed items emphasize neurological development.

How to Use This Appendix

The milestones are organized by age ranges (e.g., 0–3 months, 4–6 months). By the end of each range, most children should be able to accomplish the skills described. Roughly 25% of children will achieve them earlier, 50% will fall in the middle of the range, and the remaining 25% may reach them closer to the later end.

It's important to remember that every child develops at a unique pace. Timing is influenced by a child's interests, the opportunities they're given to explore and practice, and the degree of intentional involvement from parents or caregivers.

If a child consistently misses milestones or falls significantly behind, this may indicate underlying developmental delays. In such cases, consultation with an expert is recommended. While many families first turn to a pediatrician or medical doctor, it is also valuable to involve providers who can implement proactive, noninvasive solutions to help children get back on track—such as an upper cervical doctor or pediatric chiropractor.

0-3 Months

- **Motor Skills**:
    - Tummy time in sphinx position.
    - Excitement movements (wiggling arms and legs).
    - Opens and closes fists.
    - Brings hands to mouth.

- **Sensory and Interaction**:
    - Visually tracks and reaches for faces or toys.
    - Turns head toward noises and voices.
    - Maintains eye contact.

- **Communication**:
    - Varied cries (hungry, tired, diaper change).
    - Coos and smiles.

- **Feeding**:
    - Latches effectively.
    - Proper tongue movement and feeding suction.
    - Feeds 4-6 times per day.

4-6 Months

- **Motor Skills**:
    - Begins self-supported sitting.
    - Rolls over both ways.
    - Legs react to supported standing.
    - Transfers toys between hands.

- **Sensory and Interaction**:
  - Happy demeanor.
  - Focuses on the speaker when spoken to.
- **Communication**:
  - Consonant sounds and babbling.
- **Feeding**:
  - Opens mouth for food.
  - Begins eating solids (sticks or purees).
  - Maintains latch, tongue movement, and feeding suction.
  - Feeds 4-6 times per day.

7-9 Months

- **Motor Skills**:
  - Sits without support.
  - Moves from laying to sitting.
  - Displays cross-crawl pattern.
- **Fine Motor Skills**:
  - Develops small object dexterity.
  - Turns board book pages.
- **Sensory and Interaction**:
  - Engages in imitation play (mimicking clapping, peekaboo, hand motion songs etc).
  - Focused and attentive to the environment.
- **Communication**:
  - Syllabic babbling.
  - Basic ASL signs (e.g., more, sleep, food, milk).
- **Feeding**:
  - Holds bottle.
  - Engages in mouth mapping with food.

10-12 Months

- **Motor Skills:**
  - Pulls to stand and begins cruising.
  - Stands alone for a few seconds.

- **Fine Motor Skills:**
  - Clasps hands.
  - Demonstrates a pincer grasp (index finger and thumb grasp).
  - Places objects into large openings (like a shapes puzzle).

- **Sensory and Interaction:**
  - Enjoys familiar songs and sounds.

- **Communication:**
  - Engages in rhythmic babbling.
  - Responds to simple commands.

- **Feeding:**
  - Begins feeding self solid foods and utensil training.
  - Points to indicate wants or needs.

13-18 Months

- **Motor Skills:**
  - Walks independently.
  - Squats and regains balance.

- **Fine Motor Skills:**
  - Stacks objects.

- **Sensory and Interaction:**
  - Regular sleep schedule develops.
  - Helps with getting dressed/undressed.

- **Communication:**
  - Sound/gesture combinations.
  - Responds to familiar objects in pictures.

- Uses 5-10 words.
- **Feeding:**
  - Open cup training.
  - Eats solid foods regularly.

19-23 Months

- **Motor Skills:**
  - Basic jumping mechanics.
  - Basic running mechanics.
  - Climbs and mimics sports.

- **Fine Motor Skills:**
  - Starts drawing training.
  - Practices item stacking and puzzle work.

- **Communication:**
  - Vocabulary expands to 50 words.
  - Forms 2-word phrases.
  - Identifies body parts.
  - Understands simple instructions.

- **Cognitive Development:**
  - Listens to stories and engages with them.

24-36 Months

- **Communication:**
  - Forms 2-3 word phrases.
  - Understands concepts like "in" vs. "on."
  - 50-75% of speech is understood by others.
  - Follows 2-step directions.
  - Understands "mine" vs. "yours."
  - Answers simple "What" and "Where" questions.

- **Motor Skills**:
  - Improves running and jumping.
  - Climbs with confidence.

For More Information

For more milestones beyond 3 years (and additional detail not covered in this book), visit the American Academy of Pediatrics at healthychildren.org or consult your local Upper Cervical Doctor or Pediatric Chiropractor.

Appendix B

Specialists

Which Provider for Which Issue

This appendix provides a guide to the types of healthcare providers that can assist parents in addressing concerns in different categories of care. These recommendations help you identify which professional to consult based on your child's needs, ensuring a targeted and effective approach to their care.

Upper Cervical Chiropractor: For addressing structural misalignments in the craniocervical junction and supporting brainstem function.

Pediatric Chiropractor: For spinal alignment and neuromuscular issues impacting the nervous system.

Pediatric Neurologist: For concerns related to brain development, neurological disorders, or seizure activity.

Holistic Pediatrician: For comprehensive, integrative assessments that balance natural and medical approaches.

Functional Neurologist: For evaluations of brain function, learning disabilities, and neurological optimization.

Art or Play Therapist: For younger children struggling to express emotions or process trauma.

Functional Medicine Practitioner: For comprehensive evaluations of chemical toxicity, hormonal imbalances, and chronic illness.

Naturopathic Doctor: For toxin elimination, herbal remedies, and natural approaches to detoxification.

Environmental Testing Company: For evaluating and mitigating toxins in your home environment (e.g., mold, air quality, chemicals).

Pediatric Dietitian or Nutritionist: For guidance on balanced diets, addressing nutrient deficiencies, and managing food intolerances.

Functional Nutritionist: For tailored approaches to nutrition based on individual needs and metabolic function.

Doctor of Chinese Medicine: For incorporating plant-based remedies to support digestion, immunity, and overall health. This is a strong Eastern alternative to Western pharmaceutically based medical care.

Orthodontist or Airway Dentist: For addressing structural issues related to jaw development, airway function, and dental alignment.

Myofunctional Therapist: For supporting proper tongue, jaw, and oral development to enhance breathing and posture.

Craniosacral Therapist: For gentle adjustments of cranial bones and promoting cerebrospinal fluid flow.

Neuromuscular Therapist: For improving nerve-muscle coordination and relieving tension that impacts nervous system function.

Neurofeedback Practitioner: For using advanced technology to train the brain and improve communication pathways.

Appendix C

Resources & Research

Further Reading of Deeper Understanding

Pregnancy and Birth

- **Mama Natural: The Week-by-Week Guide to Pregnancy and Childbirth** by Genevieve Howland
  A natural, empowering approach to pregnancy and childbirth, offering week-by-week guidance and practical tips for moms-to-be.

- **The Birth Guy's Go-To Guide for New Dads; How to Support Your Partner Through Birth, Breastfeeding, and Beyond** by Brain W. Salmon, Kirsten Brunner, and Chris Pegula
  A stage-by-stage guide aimed to equip fathers with practical steps to care for their partner through pregnancy, birth, breastfeeding, and parenting.

Childhood Health and Development

- **How to Raise a Healthy Child in Spite of Your Doctor: One of America's Leading Pediatricians Puts Parents Back in Control of Their Children's Health** by Robert S. Mendelsohn
  A comprehensive guide on common health ailments and empowering parents to be primary health guides of the family.

- **Disconnected Kids: The Groundbreaking Brain Balance Program for Children with Autism, ADHD, Dyslexia, and Other Neurological Disorders** by Dr. Robert Melillo

    A guide to understanding and addressing developmental delays and neurological disorders using an integrative brain-body approach.

- **Reconnected Kids: Help Your Child Achieve Physical, Mental, and Emotional Balance** by Dr. Robert Melillo

    A step-by-step program to strengthen family relationships and support a child's neurological health.

- **The Disconnected Kids Nutrition Plan: Proven Strategies to Enhance Learning and Focus for Children with Autism, ADHD, Dyslexia, and Other Neurological Disorders** by Dr. Robert Melillo

    A practical guide to improving children's neurological health through targeted nutrition strategies.

Vaccination Decisions

- **The Vaccine Book: Making the Right Decision for Your Child** by Dr. Robert W. Sears

    A balanced and thorough resource for understanding vaccines and making informed decisions tailored to your family's needs

- **Informed Consent Action Network (ICAN) – icandecide.org**

    A resource hub dedicated to transparency in medicine, offering research, legal updates, and educational tools to help families make informed health decisions.

Further Parental Guidance

- **The On Becoming Babywise Series** by Gary Ezzo and Robert Bucknam, MD

    A comprehensive strategy to sleep training and developing a well-trained child. Books from Babywise through Teenwise for every stage of development.

Research References

1. Hamilton BE, Martin JA, Osterman MJK. Births: Provisional data for 2022. *Natl Vital Stat Rep.* 2023;72(1):1-9.
2. World Health Organization. WHO Statement on Caesarean Section Rates. Geneva: World Health Organization; 2015. Report No.: WHO/RHR/15.02. Available from: https://www.who.int/publications/i/item/WHO-RHR-15.02
3. "Incidence of Somatic Dysfunction in Healthy Newborns." *J Am Osteopath Assoc.* 2015;115(11):654-665. doi:10.7556/jaoa.2015.136.
4. El Shakankiry HM. Sleep physiology and sleep disorders in childhood. Nat Sci Sleep. 2011;3:101-114. doi:10.2147/NSS.S25689.
5. Cleveland Clinic. Recommended Amount of Sleep for Children. Cleveland Clinic Health Essentials. Published May 5, 2021. Accessed December 31, 2024. https://health.clevelandclinic.org/recommended-amount-of-sleep-for-children
6. Scime NV, Metcalfe A, Nettel-Aguirre A, Nerenberg K, Seow CH, Tough SC, Chaput KH. Breastfeeding difficulties in the first 6 weeks postpartum among mothers with chronic conditions: a latent class analysis. BMC Pregnancy Childbirth. 2023;23(1):90. doi:10.1186/s12884-023-05407-w. PMID: 36732799; PMCID: PMC9893695.
7. Centers for Disease Control and Prevention (CDC). Preventing Adverse Childhood Experiences (ACEs): Leveraging the Best Available Evidence. [Internet]. Atlanta (GA): Centers for Disease Control and Prevention; 2019 Nov [cited 2024 Jan 1]. Available from: https://www.cdc.gov/vitalsigns/aces/index.html.

About the Authors

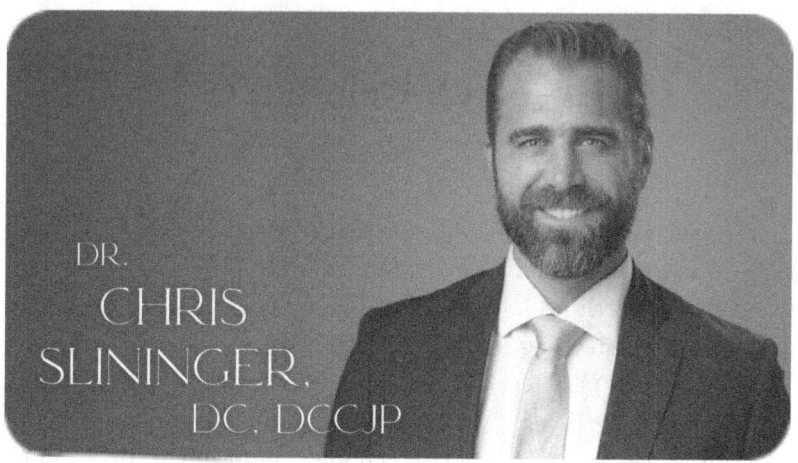

Dr. Chris Slininger has dedicated his career to helping families, leaders, and professionals protect and optimize their most valuable asset—the brain. A U.S. Army veteran and nationally recognized craniocervical specialist, his mission is to uncover and share the principles that make the body and mind thrive, equipping parents and children alike to build resilience, unlock potential, and live healthier lives.

As the owner and Clinic Director of Cerebral Chiropractic Center in St. Petersburg, Florida, Dr. Slininger works with patients facing complex neurological and developmental challenges. His practice specializes in conditions such as headaches, migraines, dizziness, brain fog, intracranial pressure, post-concussion syndrome, dysautonomia, and more—always with a root cause approach to restoring function and improving quality of life.

He also serves as the Executive Director of the Advanced Orthogonal Institute, where he trains doctors across the country in the cutting-edge technique of Advanced Orthogonal. He has served on the Board of Directors of the International Chiropractic Association's

Council on Upper Cervical Care and is the founder of Synapse Continuing Education, an organization providing cross-professional training for healthcare providers on some of the most innovative topics, procedures, and technologies in modern healthcare.

In addition to his clinical and organizational leadership, Dr. Slininger is a professional speaker with the Voices of Valor Speaking Group and teaches continuing education nationwide. Through his keynote presentations, masterclasses, and online health courses—including *Health By God's Design* and *The Eating Perfectly Masterclass*—he translates complex neuroscience into simple, practical strategies. His teaching equips audiences to build resilience, harness stress for growth, and protect brain health while pursuing success in both work and family life.

Beyond his professional achievements, Dr. Slininger's greatest joy is found at home. He and his wife, Mary, have been married for more than 15 years and are raising five children. His experiences as a husband and father not only inspire his work but also ground his writing in the practical realities of family life, giving him a unique perspective on the challenges and hopes of parents seeking the best for their children.

About the Authors

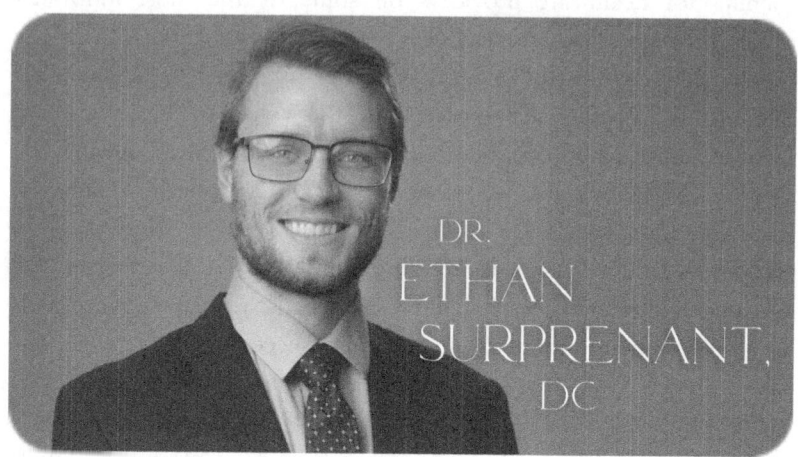

Dr. Dr. Ethan Surprenant is dedicated to helping families unlock the potential within their children by addressing the root causes of neurodevelopmental challenges. His mission is to make the principles of brain health clear and accessible so parents can confidently guide their children through each stage of growth and development.

An Upper Cervical Chiropractor with advanced training in pediatric neurodevelopment, Dr. Surprenant specializes in conditions such as ADHD, dysautonomias, POTS, sensory processing disorder, and other neurological and neurodevelopmental concerns. He completed his Doctorate of Chiropractic at Life University in Marietta, Georgia, with a focus on upper cervical care, and went on to complete training through the Advanced Orthogonal Institute as well as certification through the Holder Research Institute for Torque Release Technique. In addition, he completed The Dysautonomia Project's Provider Training, equipping him with advanced strategies for helping patients with autonomic nervous system disorders.

Dr. Surprenant serves both children and families with a neurologically based pediatric practice designed to address the unique challenges that come with pregnancy, birth, and childhood. His family-centered approach allows him to meet children and parents where they are, offering practical strategies and compassionate care.

In addition to his clinical practice, Dr. Surprenant is committed to community education. He partners with schools, parent groups, and professional organizations to share insights on neurodevelopmental health, bridging the gap between science and everyday family life.

Outside of practice, he finds fulfillment as a husband and father, which deepens his connection to the families he serves. His personal and professional experiences give him a unique ability to empathize with parents while offering hope and clarity for the road ahead.

Made in the USA
Columbia, SC
14 October 2025